YOGA Therapy for

Headache Relief

YOGA Therapy for

Headache Relief

Peter Van Houten, M.D., and Gyandev McCord, Ph.D.

Crystal Clarity Publishers
Nevada City, California

Design by C. A. Starner Schuppe
Photography by Sugar Pine Studios

ISBN: 1-56589-169-4
Printed in China
3 5 7 9 10 11 8 6 4 2

Crystal Clarity Publishers
14618 Tyler-Foote Road
Nevada City, CA 95959-8599

Phone: 800-424-1055 or 530-478-7600
Fax: 530-478-7610
E-mail: clarity@crystalclarity.com
Website: www.crystalclarity.com

Library of Congress CIP data available.

Table of Contents

Introduction *7*

A Note on the Yoga
Practices in This Book *11*

One *15* Headaches—Who *Hasn't* Had One?

Two *21* Which Kind of Headache Is It—Tension or Migraine?

Three *35* Other Causes of Headaches

Four *41* Ananda Yoga™—An Ideal Headache Treatment

Five *49* Keys to the Practice of Ananda Yoga for Headache Relief

Six *59* Ananda Yoga™ Headache Prevention Techniques

Seven *127* Additional Postures

Eight *133* Ananda Yoga™ Headache Intervention Routine

Nine *141* More You Can Do for Your Headaches

Ten *147* Summary of the Main Routine

Appendix A *152* Medical Bibliography

Appendix B *155* Additional Steps You Can Take with Ananda Yoga™

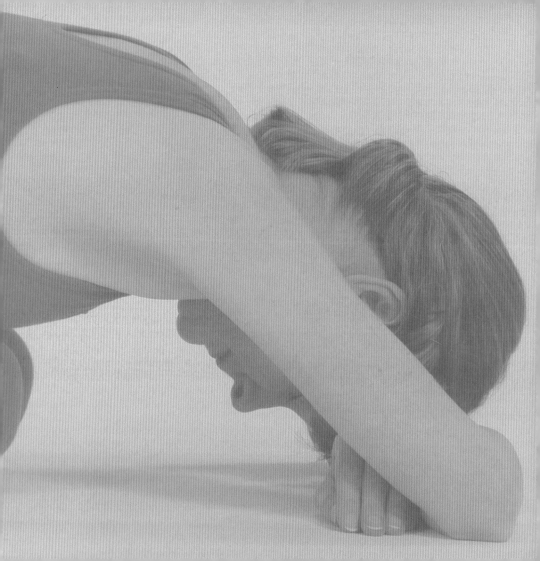

Introduction

"Sorry, but I have a headache...."

If you are a headache sufferer or know someone who is, you'll find this book a tremendous resource. Although the medical treatment of headaches has improved in recent years, you may be one of many who are unable to get adequate relief with the currently available headache medications. You may be discouraged by the high cost and side effects of the medications you are taking. Or you may simply be looking for an approach to your headaches that emphasizes wellness over medication.

In this book, you'll learn how you can dramatically affect your headaches using specific yoga postures, stretches, relaxation, deep breathing, and affirmations, as part of the well-known system of Ananda Yoga™. The yoga posture routines and other suggestions in this book are designed to blend with any of the standard medical therapies you may already be receiving.

You'll find that most physicians are already familiar with the positive effects that relaxation and stretching techniques can have on a host of medical problems, including headaches. For example, a recent study found that one commonly prescribed medication for tension headaches was really no more effective than stress management training in preventing those headaches. Another study released in 2002 that looked at migraine headaches in teenagers found that behavioral therapy might be better for treating migraine headaches than some of the standard medications. The activities suggested in this book are ones that most physicians would wholeheartedly endorse. Your health care provider may have already recommended this book or activities like this as an addition to your headache medical care.

This book offers an easy-to-understand review of the latest scientific medical evidence about headaches, including their causes, diagnoses, and treatment. You'll also learn how the ancient tradition of yoga approaches the treatment of headaches using the Ananda Yoga™ system. This is an excellent handbook with enjoyable, and highly effective, yoga routines and exercises that you can start using today. With the deep physical relaxation and serenity you'll feel with these yoga routines, along with the improvement in your headaches you'll benefit in many other ways, physically, mentally, and emotionally.

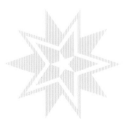

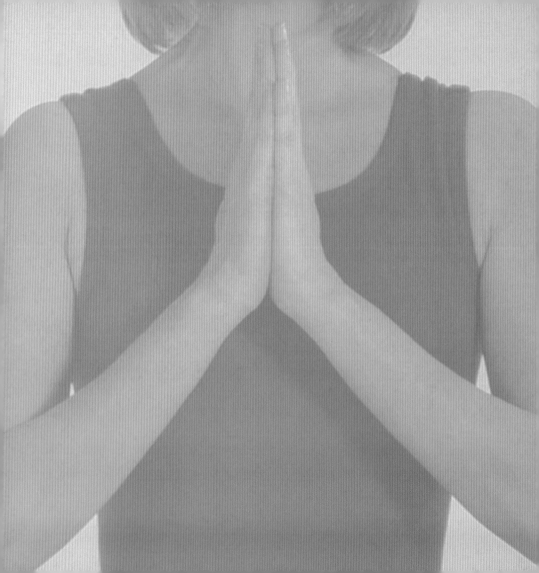

A Note on the Yoga Practices in This Book

This book is designed to blend seamlessly with the medical care you are currently receiving for your headaches. Any actual changes in your medication or treatment should, of course, be made in consultation with your health care provider.

While the exercises we present here are simple, not all yoga practices are suitable for everyone. To reduce the risk of injury, it's a good idea to consult your doctor before beginning any exercise program like this one.

Obviously, the instructions and advice in this book are not intended as substitutes for medical counsel from your health care advisor.

The therapeutic approach in this book is intended to benefit a wide range of people suffering from headaches, and for most people it is an excellent starting point. To get the greatest therapeutic benefit, it's even better to work individually with a qualified yoga instructor who can draw upon a broader range of yoga therapy techniques and tailor your program to your own unique needs and abilities. Bear in mind, however, that although yoga therapy often has immediate effects, usually it is not a "quick fix"; rather, it is a gradual route to enduring harmony on all levels of your being. For more information about Ananda Yoga and actual personal instruction, look in Appendix B: "Additional Steps You Can Take with Ananda Yoga."

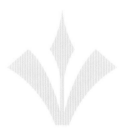

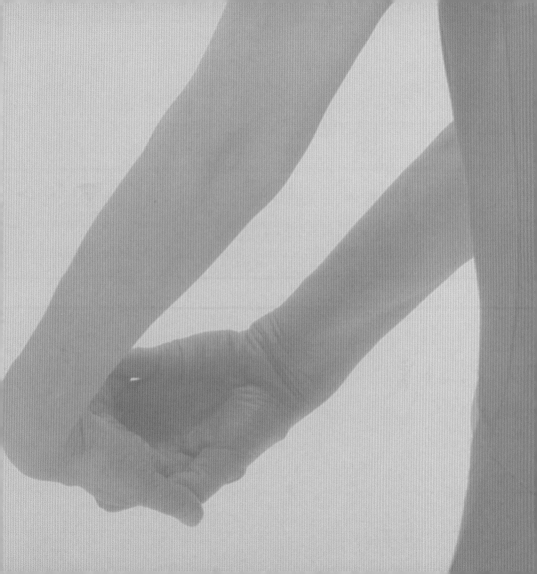

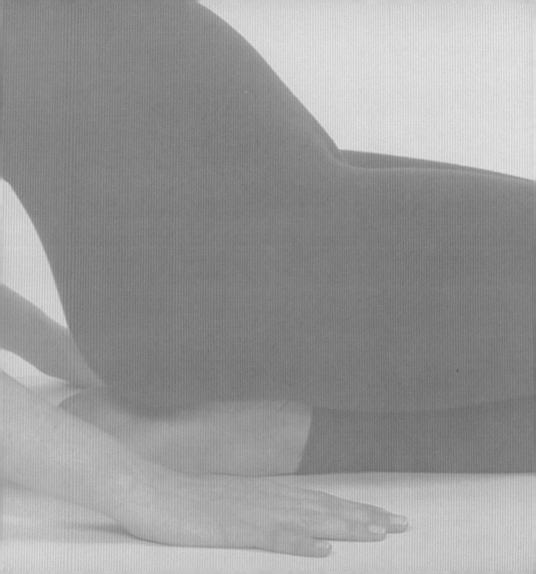

Chapter One

Headaches—Who *Hasn't* Had One?

An Epidemic Problem

Almost everyone has experienced a bad headache at some time. Fortunately, for most people, it's an occasional problem usually associated with a case of the flu or a particularly stressful day. It's not surprising that roughly half of the U.S. population have had a severe headache at least once in their lives.

However, you may be one of the millions of people who have had a serious problem with recurrent headaches. In fact, headaches are one of the most common reasons people visit their doctor. More than 5% of adults are currently receiving medical care related to headaches and about 15% have had a serious problem with headaches at some point during their lifetimes.

If you suffer from chronic headaches, you already know how disabling they can be. On a national scale, the costs for treating headaches are enormous. In a typical year, Americans take over 15,000 tons of aspirin for headaches as well as countless truckloads of ibuprofen and acetaminophen (Tylenol). Untold millions of hours of work are missed yearly because of headache-related problems. Migraine headaches alone are thought to result in up to 17 billion dollars worth of lost worker productivity yearly!

Not surprisingly, chronic headaches over time tend to undermine the sufferer's emotional and physical health in general. Ultimately, even close social relationships can deteriorate as a result of recurrent headaches. For example, those with migraine headaches are three times more likely to develop depression than those without migraines.

Many Headache Sufferers Find Little Relief

Many people with significant recurrent headaches never seek medical care for diagnosis and possible treatment. You or someone you know may be among the millions who simply suffer. Some are unable to find a doctor with whom they feel comfortable, while others simply can't afford medical care. Many headache sufferers are dissatisfied with standard medical treatments they've received in the past and don't want to go back. A surprising number of headache sufferers are convinced that finding an effective, side-effect-free treatment is a hopeless task. Any physician will tell you that treating chronic headaches can be a frustrating experience for both doctor and patient. Every conscientious physician wants affordable, safe, and effective headache relief for all his patients and is often faced with inadequate treatment options.

If you've been treated for headaches, you may have experienced firsthand some of the problems related to medications used in treating headaches, including simply not enough pain relief. Or you may have gotten some unpleasant side effects from your medication. Quite understandably, you may also worry about the potential negative effects of taking a headache medication regularly over many years. Frankly, many people are just tired of being dependent on medication in order to live free of headaches. Some rebel at the extremely high cost of prescription medications for headaches or find that they simply can't afford them.

This book offers you alternatives that will complement any standard medical care for headaches you are already receiving. Even if you've found a medication that works well for you, you may still want a more natural, preventive approach to headache treatment as a way to be less dependent on medication. One of the goals of this Ananda Yoga program is to gradually lessen your need for medication, and possibly make drugs unnecessary altogether. Our approach to headache management uses a special sequence of yoga postures and exercises that can help you prevent recurrent headaches or ease a headache that is already in progress. Based on the well-known Ananda Yoga system, these exercises emphasize relaxation, stretching, deep breathing, and positive affirmation to break the headache cycle.

Often, physicians would like to suggest these types of relaxation exercises and stretches for many different medical problems, including headaches. But, in reality, few doctors actually have a well-rounded program that they can easily offer to their patients, or the extra time they need to teach it. You'll find this book a simple to use, step-by-step guide that will teach you a set of yoga exercises that is very effective for headaches. This is a medication-free way to treat your headaches that is both easy and enjoyable.

This book covers the role of Ananda Yoga in headache treatment and also the traditional "yoga theory" behind it. It also reviews the current medical understanding of the causes of headaches and the latest medical treatments. You'll learn the physiology behind the effectiveness of these yoga stretches. If you're currently being treated for headaches, you may want to share this book with your physician, who may have other patients who want to explore non-drug therapies as an additional aid. Ananda Yoga is a powerful tool that complements any standard medical treatment by treating the underlying mental and physiological origins of headaches.

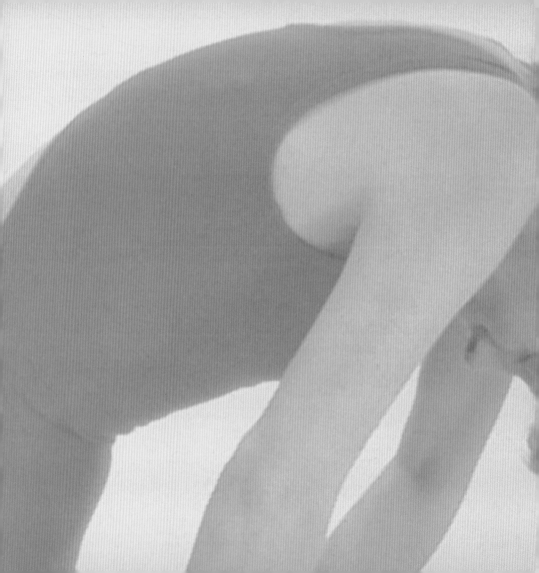

Chapter Two

Which Kind of Headache Is It— Tension or Migraine?

Two main types of headaches—migraine and tension headaches—account for about 90% of all chronic headaches. Let's start with two case examples that will give you a feel for what these common headaches can be like.

Case #1—Elaine: Disabled by Her Headaches

Elaine is in her mid-50s and has just received the promotion of her dreams to a top managerial position at the insurance firm where she has worked for years. With her new duties have come much more responsibility and stress. Her mild migraine headaches, which she'd been having only once or twice a year, are hitting her three times a week and are unbelievably painful. When she first started having migraines forty years ago as a teenager, they were occasionally this bad, but by her twenties they'd almost gone away. Elaine's headaches had stayed pretty mild until recently. Now, every day when she wakes up, she's filled with apprehensive thoughts: "Will I have a killer headache today?"

Just before each headache starts, Elaine notices that her vision is briefly peppered with bright flashes of light. She also has trouble concentrating. Within minutes the actual headache begins, pounding and intense, usually behind her left eye. Elaine is terribly nauseated and vomits at least several times uncontrollably. Any noise or light is annoying, so she usually ends up in bed, in darkness and quiet. In the last month, she has had to abruptly leave three different meetings with important clients because of headaches like this. She's used up a year's worth of sick leave in four months and her most recent headache lasted two days—a record for her. Her boss has started warning her about her performance.

Elaine's doctor has recently prescribed a number of different medications for her headaches; they work well sometimes, but only about half the time. Elaine's even tried taking several different medications daily that are designed to prevent her headaches. So far, they either haven't helped or the medications themselves made her feel terrible. Worst of all, she's had to stop the hormone replacement therapy prescribed for her menopause symptoms because she realized that her estrogen pills were making her headaches even worse. Now she has headaches *and* hot flashes! Elaine is feeling desperate. Her doctor is sympathetic, but out of ideas; he's arranged for her to see a specialist but her first visit is months away, because the specialist's schedule is full. Even the stress reduction therapy suggested by her doctor is out of her reach financially, since it's not covered by her insurance. She doesn't know what to do next. Elaine has classic migraine headaches.

Case # 2—David: A College Student Worried about His Headaches

David is a young, athletic, and very healthy student in his third year of college. It's final exam time and he's been putting in very long days and nights studying at the library. He's not sleeping too well and is very worried about how he will do on his exams this year. David is particularly anxious about scoring well since his guidance counselor has warned him that he needs to improve his grades if he wants to go to graduate school.

On top of all this pressure, David has started having headaches. They are like a tight band around his head and tend to come on late in the day. Even his scalp hurts sometimes. Taking a couple of ibuprofen was working fine—at first. Now, nothing seems to help, and his headaches are starting to worry him. At the student heath clinic last week, the nurse told him it was "just tension" and "not to worry about it." But David's getting frightened that maybe something is really wrong and that's why he has headaches. It's getting hard for him to study because as soon as he gets a headache, he starts to worry that it's really caused by something serious, like a brain tumor. He doesn't know what to do. David is having tension headaches.

Neither Elaine's nor David's story is unusual. Fortunately for them and the many millions of headache sufferers like them, there are proven yoga techniques that Elaine and David could start practicing to help their headaches right away—techniques that would complement the medication they take. The focus of this book is to teach anyone with recurrent headaches how to use the highly regarded Ananda Yoga system. This system's approach to yoga emphasizes relaxation, stretching, breathing, and positive affirmation—powerful tools for overcoming a headache.

But before we say more about how to solve your problem with headaches using Ananda Yoga, let's explore medical science's latest discoveries about headaches and their treatment.

The Two Common Types of Headaches

There are literally dozens of different causes for recurrent headaches. The vast majority of headaches, however, are either migraine headaches or tension headaches. We'll discuss these two common types in detail since they account for almost all recurrent headaches; some of the less frequent causes will be reviewed in the next section. Because these two types are overwhelmingly the most common cause of recurrent headaches, most headaches are diagnosed based solely on a person's symptoms and physical examination. Only rarely do headaches require extensive and expensive testing, such as a brain MRI or CT scan.

Migraines

Amazingly, about 10% of people may have some form of migraine headaches, just like Elaine in our example above. Close to half of all the recurrent headaches that are evaluated by physicians turn out to be a type of migraine or a mixture of migraine and tension headaches. The tendency toward migraines is often inherited and affects women three times more often than men. As many as one out of five women may experience migraines. Migraine headaches usually begin in childhood or early adulthood, but some women develop them only after menopause. Most people average about 12 attacks a year, but some individuals may have migraines much more frequently than this. Fewer than half of those with migraines are ever "formally" diagnosed by a physician as having migraines.

A migraine may start quite abruptly and unexpectedly. The actual headache part of the migraines may be preceded by symptoms such as seeing bright flashes of light or geometric patterns, or feelings of confusion. Some sufferers have weakness or tingling in an arm or leg, or even have difficulty speaking prior to their headache. Any pre-headache symptoms are called an "aura," and usually last less than 30 minutes. Typically the aura symptoms end with the start of the headache. Many people with migraines don't have these aura symptoms. During a migraine, the headache is often one-sided, but can involve the whole head and typically has a throbbing or pounding quality. Exercise tends to make the pain worse. The pain can be severe and can last just a few hours or for days. A migraine episode often involves many additional annoying symptoms, such as nausea with vomiting and extreme sensitivity to light and noise. Sufferers may have all or only a few of these symptoms with a migraine attack. For example, some migraine sufferers have migraines that involve only the nausea symptoms without any real headache—migraine symptoms are highly individual!

Inside the Brain during a Migraine

Our understanding of the actual events that occur in the brain during a migraine headache has improved in recent years. It seems likely that an imbalance in the brain's neurotransmitters deep inside the brain begins a whole cascade of events, which rapidly result in a migraine headache. Neurotransmitters are the chemical messengers that the cells in the brain use to communicate with one another. When there is a specific type of imbalance in these neurotransmitters a headache can result. It's thought that the headache pain itself is actually caused by inflammation, irritation, and swelling of the blood vessels in the brain. All these inflammatory changes in the brain appear to be initiated by changes in neurotransmitters, with the neurotransmitter called serotonin most often implicated.

Triggers for Migraines

Many things can precipitate a migraine. Psychological stress or emotional upsets are common triggers. Some women may have migraines only around the time of their menstrual period which are most likely triggered by hormonal changes. Foods such as red wine, certain cheeses, nuts, and chocolate are also known triggers for some people. A few food additives like

MSG (monosodium glutamate) or those found in processed meats can set off a migraine. A change in sleep patterns, weather changes, high altitude, bright or flickering lights, and strong odors or fumes can bring on migraines as well. Women who start on estrogen therapy after menopause may develop migraines as a consequence of their therapy, and lowering the dose of estrogen may offer a simple solution in those cases. Some people develop "rebound" migraine headaches from taking pain relievers like ibuprofen too frequently; their headaches start whenever they miss their usual dose!

Medication treatment for a rapidly developing migraine attack can involve simply taking ibuprofen if the migraine is mild. There are also newer prescription medications, including the ergotamine derivative DHE and a class of medications called the "triptans." Imitrex, Zomig, Maxalt, Axert, and Amerge are some of the brand names of triptans commonly prescribed. These newer medications are often successful in stopping a migraine by affecting the brain's neurotransmitters directly. They can be given by tablet, nasal spray, or injection, depending on the particular drug. Caffeine can also be useful in breaking the course of a migraine and can be found combined with other pain relievers in tablet form. For those with frequent migraines or those who have severe, disabling migraines, there are also preventive prescription medications that are taken daily and are mentioned further on in this book. Even riboflavin, which is vitamin B2, and the herb feverfew have been shown to be promising in preventing migraines when taken regularly.

Relaxation techniques, biofeedback, and autosuggestion have also been shown to be of help in the prevention of migraines. This is where Ananda Yoga adds a range of effective techniques for inducing a relaxation response, with its use of affirmations, gentle stretches, and other proven methods for calming the tense mind and body.

Tension Headaches

Tension[1] headaches are, as you might guess, the most common type of headache, affecting nearly every-

[1] In the medical profession, this kind of headache is currently called a *"tension type headache"* rather than the older, more common term *"tension headache."* This newer term is used to emphasize that these headaches are caused not only by "psychological stress" or "muscle contraction," as the words *"tension headache"* might imply, but by additional factors, as we'll discuss in this chapter. For the remainder of this book, however, we'll use the more familiar term "tension headache" to refer to this type of headache.

one at least once during a time of particular stress. About half of the people who seek out medical help for recurrent headaches have this type of headache, sometimes in combination with a migraine. Our college student David didn't need to worry about a more serious cause for his recurrent headaches. The tension and stress of today's non-stop, "multi-tasking" lifestyle is often the chief culprit behind tension headaches.

The pain from a tension headache can be as severe as that of a migraine headache but it is usually described as "band-like" and aching; typically it involves both sides of the head. The pain will be dull and fairly steady. Unlike with a migraine, exercising may actually help a tension headache. Some people experiencing this kind of headache also have neck stiffness, with pain at the back of the head that seems to radiate to the front, or forehead. Tension headaches tend to come on slowly over hours and may persist for days, or even months!

Inside the Brain during a Tension Headache

It used to be thought that the pain in a tension headache was caused solely by muscle tension in the scalp and neck strangling off the normal blood circulation to the scalp with resulting pain. We now understand that, in addition to increased muscular tension as a potential cause, there are changes in the brain's neurotransmitters and blood vessels that may contribute as well. There can be a buildup of specific chemical irritants and an accompanying inflammation in the scalp muscles that result in headache pain. The tenderness and pain in the scalp and neck is often out of proportion to any muscular tension present. Sometimes the person's scalp will even become extremely tender to the touch. It's interesting to note that physicians now feel that migraines and tension headaches may be caused by somewhat similar changes in the brain's neurotransmitters and their causes are possibly more related to each other than was once thought.

Triggers for Tension Headaches

Anxiety, depression, life stress, missed meals, sleep deprivation, and exposure to cigarette smoke are all common triggers for tension headaches. Poor posture, sitting in one position for long periods while working at a desk, or being a sedentary "couch potato" also predisposes one to this form of headache.

Treating Tension Headaches

The usual medication treatment for a tension headache once it's in progress is a mild pain reliever, like ibuprofen or acetaminophen (Tylenol). For prevention of tension headaches, neck muscle stretches and scalp massage can be helpful. Since emotional stress is often a key trigger, working with relaxation techniques is often beneficial. When significant depression and anxiety are present, it's sometimes simplest to treat these conditions directly and see if this doesn't alleviate the recurrent headaches.

Ananda Yoga is an ideal way of treating tension headaches, because it works with muscular stretches, relaxation, and positive affirmations. All these techniques act directly on the underlying cause of tension headaches—and in a way that promotes a profound sense of well-being and calm.

Chapter Three

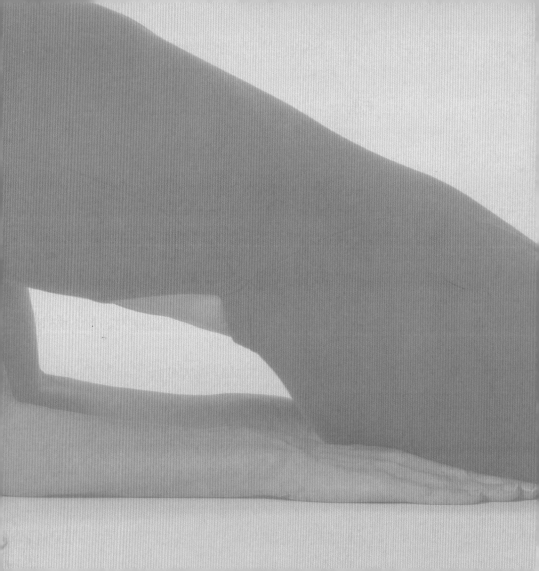

Other Causes of Headaches

About 90% of the chronic headaches that physicians evaluate turn out to be tension or migraine headaches, but the remaining 10% have a broad range of causes. Fortunately only a few of them are serious.

One commonly held misconception concerning headaches is that they are caused by "eyestrain." However, new glasses are almost never the cure—visual problems are a surprisingly rare cause of chronic headaches.

Both tension and migraine headaches are sometimes misdiagnosed as sinus headaches. However, sinus-related headaches are not that common and almost always include facial pain directly over the sinuses, along with other sinus symptoms, such as a constant runny nose.

Many medications can cause headaches as an unfortunate side effect. Some of the biggest culprits are the medicines that are used to treat high blood pressure, hormone therapy for women, and oral contraceptives.

Abruptly stopping one's coffee consumption may cause a "caffeine withdrawal" headache severe enough to land the sufferer in the Emergency Room! Dehydration, even fairly mild, is another common headache cause. "Am I drinking enough non-caffeinated fluid?" should be one of the first questions you ask yourself at the onset of a headache. Lastly, many viral illnesses will cause a headache as part of their symptoms, as every flu sufferer can attest.

As you can see, most of the less common causes of recurrent headaches have other symptoms which accompany the headache and make a diagnosis simpler.

A Headache Is Rarely a Sign of a Serious Problem

Fortunately, chronic headaches are only rarely a sign of an underlying serious condition. Those with chronic headaches who are evaluated by a physician have less than a 1% chance of having something truly worrisome, such as a brain tumor. In our case example in the last chapter, there was really little chance that David's headaches were caused by something as bad as he feared.

If you're worried, having your headaches evaluated by a physician is a good, practical step for your own peace of mind. While migraines and tension headaches can be excruciatingly painful, and even disabling, you can at least relieve yourself of the stress that comes from thinking that something potentially life-threatening is wrong with you. And less stress is, after all, the beginning of the solution to your headaches.

Some Other Uncommon Causes and Types of Chronic Headaches

- Post-concussion headache from a head injury
- Brain tumor
- Brain aneurysm—a chronically distended blood vessel section in the brain
- Trigeminal neuralgia—a painfully inflamed facial nerve
- TMJ disorder—"jaw joint" pain
- Drug abuse
- Subdural hematoma—a pocket of blood in the space between the brain and the skull, typically after a head injury
- Temporal arteritis—a chronically inflamed scalp artery at the temple
- Cluster headaches—headaches that occur in "clustered" time periods
- Carbon monoxide poisoning—most commonly from poorly ventilated stoves or car exhaust
- Significant untreated high blood pressure
- Brain abscess—pocket of infection in the brain
- Stroke
- Lyme disease—brain infection caused by the bite of a certain infected tick
- Sleep apnea—episodes of breathing obstruction during sleep, causing oxygen deprivation.

What Symptoms Should Be Evaluated?

Although the vast majority of headaches have a benign cause, occasionally headaches are, indeed, a warning of something more serious. Physicians become concerned when a severe, chronic headache is persistent, or is worsening—particularly if it is localized to one area. A headache with a rapid increase in frequency is also of concern, particularly if the initial episode was within the last six months.

Severe headaches that are accompanied by a high fever or are described as "the worst headache I've ever had" should receive prompt medical attention. Chronic headaches that are associated with personality changes or other neurological changes, such as difficulty speaking or weakness or tingling in an arm or leg, can signal something more serious. Headaches that are accompanied by a loss of coordination or headaches that awaken one from sleep should be investigated. One good rule of thumb: a physician should evaluate any chronic headache that begins after age fifty.

As you can see, there are, fortunately, only a few situations that warrant intensive medical evaluation. Most headaches can be evaluated in a physician's office with just a thorough physical exam and careful review of a person's symptoms.

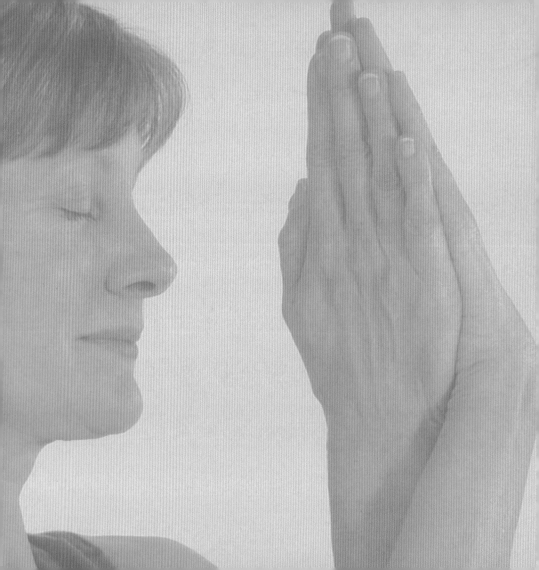

Chapter Four

Ananda Yoga—An Ideal Headache Treatment

Although medical treatment is available for both tension and migraine headaches, these medications may prove unacceptable. The medications for migraine headaches particularly can have unpleasant side effects or are inconsistently effective. If you have migraine headaches, you may have already tried many medications without adequate relief. Also, many migraine sufferers revolt at the thought of an entire life of taking medication daily attempting to prevent their migraines and still never knowing when their next headache will hit. Migraine headache medication can be so blindingly expensive that many people find they simply can't afford these treatments. Even taking ibuprofen frequently for tension headaches is not without risk—bleeding from the stomach can occur and, much more rarely, kidney damage.

Happily, there are other therapies that any physician can wholeheartedly recommend. Here is where Ananda Yoga enters the picture—it's safe, side-effect free, enjoyable, and has many benefits beyond just treating and preventing headaches. Interestingly, even insurance companies have begun to recommend yoga therapy and similar techniques as preventive treatments for a host of chronic medical ailments including cardiac disease. Their interest, of course, is to lower medical costs by eliminating the need for expensive medications and surgery. The Ananda Yoga headache prevention and treatment program outlined in the following chapters is an excellent way to begin actively taking control over your headaches.

What makes Ananda Yoga unique is that it works in three different ways to assist in headache prevention and treatment:

1.) The postures involve beneficial, tension-relieving, gentle stretching, and because they are done meditatively, they also promote deep relaxation.

2.) Because each yoga posture is done with an affirmation, it helps realign our thought patterns to allow for headache-free living. Affirmations also help release mental tensions and stress, which are common causes for headaches.

3.) The breathing exercises done as part of Ananda Yoga also help deepen the level of relaxation, using the intimate link between breathing and mental and physical relaxation.

Traditional yoga postures by themselves are just beginning to be studied scientifically and the results, though promising, are limited to just a handful of studies. However, with the unique approach to yoga postures used in Ananda Yoga, we are applying several additional techniques—specifically that of affirmation and a meditative approach—to the practice of yoga that have been very well researched and have been shown to be helpful in a wide variety of illnesses.

Stretching

These yoga postures are highly effective yet safe stretches for the neck and upper back—key areas that need to be kept flexible to prevent tension headaches. Physicians recommend that their patients with tension headaches regularly do neck and back stretches to help prevent their headaches. These same stretches can also be used to relieve a tension headache that is in progress. While many types of neck stretches would be adequate for headache prevention and treatment, the problem is that most people won't do them regularly enough to get any real benefit. The Ananda Yoga system offers a balanced set of neck stretches that are safe, beneficial, and pleasant to do so that a regular practice is easier to keep up.

Relaxation and Stress Management

As you've seen, both migraine headaches and tension headaches are made worse by stress and emotional upset. Learning to consciously relax—the real focus of these yoga postures—is an excellent means of stress management. Meditative relaxation has been extensively studied and proven to be beneficial in preventing both migraine and tension headaches. In one recent study on the treatment of tension headaches, it was shown that after six months of treatment, an anti-depressant (a typical preventive medication for this type of headache) and stress management therapy were about equally beneficial in giving headache relief. The stress management was, of course, side-effect free.

For over thirty years, it's been known that the body has what is called a "relaxation reaction" to a meditative practice like Ananda Yoga. During this meditative state, the "fight and flight" part of our autonomic nervous system is quieted, and the "rest and repose" portion is emphasized. Automatically, in a meditative state, blood pressure decreases, the heart rate slows, as does respiration rate and oxygen consumption—all signs of deepening relaxation. Even blood levels of stress hormones begin to lower with a regular meditative practice such as Ananda Yoga offers.

As part of this deep internal relaxation, there is relaxation of your muscles as well. Particularly for tension headaches, this is highly beneficial. For example, it's been shown that in meditative relaxation the forehead muscles spontaneously relax. When under stress, many people unconsciously tighten specific muscles, particularly in their neck, face, and shoulders, which predisposes them to tension headaches.

These deeply relaxing postures help release this defensive muscular armoring so that the muscles can stay relaxed and flexible. The breathing exercises included here help to further deepen the relaxation effect. Someone who is actually in the middle of a tension headache or is having a headache that is a mixed migraine and tension headache may find that practicing these Ananda Yoga therapies lessens the pain considerably and shortens its duration, too.

Affirmation

A tremendous amount of solid research has shown that affirmation, or autosuggestion, is beneficial in many different illnesses. Autogenic training, which is very well studied and understood, is one type of therapy that takes advantage of the positive effects of affirmation. Before 1950, when many fewer medication treatments for illness existed, affirmation or autosuggestion was used more widely, but by about 1970 interest in this approach had virtually disappeared as hundreds of new and effective drugs were developed.

Recently, we've seen a resurgence of interest in affirmations or autosuggestion as an effective and safe tool for promoting good health, particularly for diseases where medication doesn't work well.

Affirmation, an essential companion to the physical postures in Ananda Yoga, is a bridge between the purely physical components contributing to your headache, and the mindset, or attitudes, which in part trigger the cascade of events resulting in a headache.

The mind-body connection denied by medical science a few short decades ago is now the starting point for a truly complete treatment of chronic headaches. Yoga has long understood what science is now arduously discovering through exhaustive study: our "thought body" tremendously influences our physical body.

Now let's move on to the actual practice of Ananda Yoga and you'll see the "yoga theory" behind these exercises. You'll learn the key yoga concepts that can be part of your headache therapy.

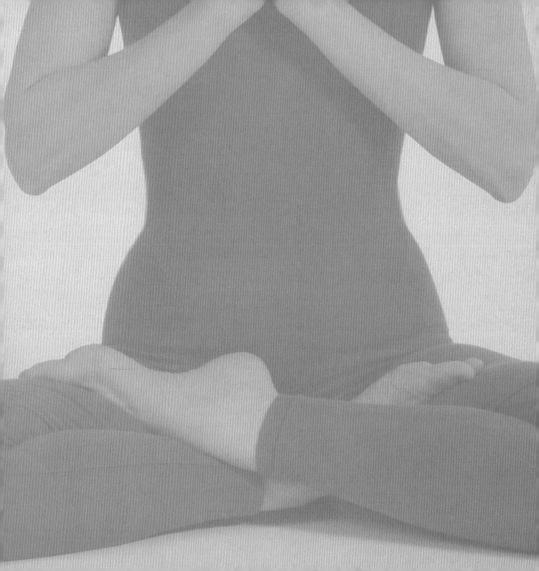

Chapter Five

Keys to the Practice of Ananda Yoga for Headache Relief

Now that we've reviewed headaches and their treatment from the standard medical perspective, let's look at headaches from the perspective of traditional yoga, the broad and ancient science of which the postures form but a small part. Yoga views health in terms of the workings of subtle energy and thought rather than just body physiology, and it's important to understand how these aspects are related.

For centuries, science has viewed matter as being composed of small particles called atoms. However, just within the last hundred years, scientists have found that these solid-appearing atoms are not solid at all; they are composed of packets of energy. Therefore, energy, not solid matter, is the real building block of our universe. Trees, rocks, water, our bodies, even the air itself—all are simply different "holding patterns" of energy.

For thousands of years traditional yoga has said much more: all energy, and hence all matter, is composed of and sustained by an even subtler form of energy, an *intelligent* energy. In Sanskrit, this subtle energy, or "life-force," is called *prana*. (Sanskrit is the language of ancient India, where yoga was developed thousands of years ago.) From the yogic perspective, prana (prah'-nah) serves as the foundation for our physical bodies; it also governs all bodily functions, maintains wellness, and promotes healing. It even affects—and is affected by—our thinking. This subtle life-force is the key to the body/mind connection so often discussed today. Although prana is not yet recognized by medical science, many traditional healing methods, including acupuncture, are designed to influence this life-force directly to promote health and wellness.

Yoga says that ill health results when the flow of prana or life-force is blocked or out of harmony. Tension headaches, for example, could be said to result from prana chronically blocked or trapped in the neck and shoulders. Or, when the life-force or prana that governs the production of neurotransmitters in the brain is out of harmony, migraine headaches could result.

Yoga offers many techniques that help unblock prana and restore its harmonious flow; the physical yoga positions (*asanas*) are the most visible of these. Asana (aah'-sah-nah) actually means "physical posture" in Sanskrit. There are many important physical benefits from stretching and relaxation; however, the greatest value of the yoga postures lies in their ability to promote and harmonize the free flow of life-force in the body.

In fact, any bodily position affects the flow of subtle energy. You can easily experience this yourself: sit up straight, take several deep breaths, smile, and lift your gaze slightly upward. Notice how you feel. Now slouch into your chair, round your spine, frown, and look downward. It's the same body as a moment ago, but you feel different—physically and mentally. Why? It's primarily the life-force. The first position encouraged the free, upward flow of energy—which yoga says is connected with feelings of happiness—whereas the second inhibited it, and even promoted a downward flow.

Similarly, each asana has a specific effect on your prana, and through it, your state of mind and health. Of course, yoga postures are not magic pills; their effects are usually quite subtle unless one goes beyond a merely physical practice of the yoga postures. (More on this in a moment.) Nevertheless, through asanas and other yoga techniques, you can work directly to harmonize your life-force.

This is the heart of Ananda Yoga, and it is not nearly so esoteric as it may seem. However, working extensively with the life-force requires training and experience beyond the scope of this book, so we will introduce you to Ananda Yoga practice in a way that will feel more familiar to you.

General Principles for Practicing Ananda Yoga

On the physical level of the practice, always move your body gracefully, with sensitive, conscious awareness. When doing the asanas, strive for comfort and relaxation, not outward achievement. This is not an athletic competition. Honor your limitations; strain brings tension and even injury, not harmony.

On the mental level, immerse your mind in the attitudes promoted by the postures. Try to *feel* those attitudes. Here the affirmations are especially helpful, for they are designed to reinforce the specific mental and energetic effects that the physical asanas promote.

The spiritual level is especially important. Whatever you wish to call it—soul, Self, light, divine essence, God—each of us knows intuitively that we have a higher reality than the body and personality. The entire science of yoga is designed to bring you into alignment with your own higher reality.

Therefore, do the postures with a feeling of ever-increasing harmony with that reality. This is the subtlest aspect of the practice, but it is not mysterious. It is you! Increasing your attunement with it will do more to harmonize the flow of life-force than anything else you can do.

Re-establishing wellness is a gradual process, but experience with yoga over millennia has shown that, for those who persevere in their practice, greater harmony and well-being will always result.

Keys to Practicing Affirmation

It is well known that affirmations can play a powerful role in wellness. These statements of higher truths help "re-program" the subconscious mind by changing harmful habits of thought into helpful habits. More importantly, they help us attune our minds with natural states of relaxation, health, harmony, and vitality—and above all, with our divine essence.

Ananda Yoga offers specific asana/ affirmation pairs designed so that each reinforces the benefits of the other. To do this effectively, however, the asana must be done without strain, and the affirmation must be used with concentration and feeling as you hold the physical position. Practice the affirmation silently, without moving tongue or lips, and without tensing the vocal cords as if to speak.

Concentration is vital to success in anything. Just as the focused beam of a laser is more powerful than the dispersed rays of an ordinary light bulb, a focused mind will charge your words with power. If at first your mind is scattered, then repeat the affirmation aloud to gain focus.

Once your mind is focused, repeat the affirmation silently—over and over, with ever more concentration—to direct your efforts inwardly to the core of your being.

Feeling, too, is vital for affirmation. Mechanical repetition brings minimal results. Instead, strive to *experience* the quality suggested by the affirmation. When affirming an enthusiastic attitude, *be* enthusiastic. When affirming peacefulness, strive to *feel* increasing peace as you repeat the affirmation.

It may take practice to get beyond the thought that you're "just pretending," but remember: affirmation is not about trying to convince yourself of anything; it's about attuning your mind to a higher octave of your own being. You already *are* that—you just need to improve your knowing. This takes concentration, feeling, and whole-hearted participation. When you realize that your state of mind is within your control, your affirmations will gain tremendous power.

Practical Guidelines for Ananda Yoga Practice

1. Before practicing the Main Routine described in this book, wait at least three hours after a large meal, and 1-2 hours after a snack. (The Basic Five exercises described below can be practiced anytime.)

2. Practice in a warm, quiet, well-ventilated place, out of direct sunlight.

3. Wear stretchy, or loose, comfortable clothing.

4. If a posture is uncomfortable for you, modify it to suit your body rather than trying to force your body into some "ideal" position. (For many of the postures in this book, easier modifications are also described.) Even if you can do the pose, but your body trembles with exertion, your efforts will be counterproductive. The fastest route to success is to find a modification that matches your current abilities. Use props (cushions, blankets, etc.) as needed to accomplish this.

$5.$ Honor the cautions given for each pose.

$6.$ Keep your breath flowing easily at all times. Holding your breath or ragged breathing while in a posture is usually a sign of strain, which draws you away from relaxation and harmony.

$7.$ Practice the postures meditatively, with a sense of patient, relaxed, alert, inward awareness, and complete involvement with what you are doing.

$8.$ When ending your practice with deep relaxation, remove your glasses or contact lenses.

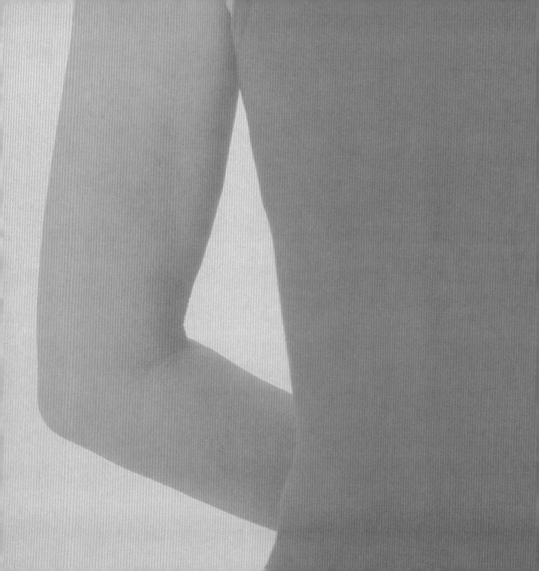

Chapter Six

Ananda Yoga Headache Prevention Techniques

Yoga Techniques for Headaches

We offer two basic sets of yoga techniques for headache treatment:

Main Routine—a basic sequence for relieving chronic tension and improving posture to prevent tension headaches, with gentle inverted poses (asanas) to help counter the tendency to develop migraines. The entire routine takes less than 20 minutes. The Main Routine should be avoided when a migraine headache is in progress because exercise may aggravate it. Instead, use the Intervention Routine outlined in the next chapter.

Intervention Routine—a short sequence that can help relieve the discomfort of a tension headache or combination migraine-tension headache in progress.

How to Use the Routines

For some of the exercises, you will need one or two firm blankets and perhaps a straight-backed chair and yoga strap. A long sock or an old necktie can be substituted for the strap. Use the exercises as follows:

Week 1:
Practice the Basic Five (exercises 4-8 on pages 76-95) at least twice daily—4 to 5 times daily for severe cases—with one of those times being just before going to bed at night. Each practice takes 6 or 7 minutes.

Weeks 2-3:
Practice the Basic Five at least twice daily, with one of those times being just before going to bed at night. On three days of each week, substitute the Main Routine for one practice of the Basic Five.

Weeks 4-5:
Practice as in weeks 2-3, but begin to hold some of the positions for longer periods. Exercises 1, 8, 9, and 12 of the Main Routine are particularly good to practice longer than the suggested guidelines.

After Week 5:

Practice as in weeks 4-5, but add to the Main Routine one or more of the postures described in the next chapter, "Additional Postures." The Ear-Closing Pose is especially beneficial.

At some point, depending on the particulars of your own body, you may have made enough progress to be able to cut back to a "maintenance level." When this happens, you can practice just the Basic Five, once or twice each day, plus a balanced routine of yoga postures three times a week. See Appendix B "Additional Steps You Can Take with Ananda Yoga" for guidance on creating a complete Ananda Yoga routine.

Throughout these routines, whenever possible—and especially in relaxation poses such as the Child Pose and Corpse Pose—close your

eyes and gently turn them upward, as though you were gazing softly at a point a few feet in front of you, slightly above the horizon. Don't try to see anything, and don't turn your eyes so far upward that they feel strained. Relax your eyes in this position as though they were being drawn naturally toward that point. This position of the eyes will become comfortable with practice. It is a classical yoga technique that gently nudges your awareness toward a state of relaxed concentration and joy.

Correct Standing Posture

Those who suffer from tension headaches often have unhealthy standing posture. For those individuals, even the simplest postural adjustments can make a significant difference. For this reason, we will focus on just a few of the many aspects of healthy posture. Practice them throughout your day.

Perhaps the most common cause of neck and shoulder tension is a slouching posture. (figure 1, page 65) Teenagers often slouch, as do many of us who work at a computer. As a result, we may carry poor posture into the rest of our day: when we stand, the pelvis stays tucked under and shifted forward, knees may be locked, the chin juts forward, the shoulders round, and the chest is caved in. No wonder the body is unhappy.

Another cause of headaches is "head forward posture": instead of sitting comfortably in line with a straight spine, the head rides way ahead of the rest of the body, dragging the body along behind it. This is common in individuals who are chronically in a hurry, and in persons who rely primarily on the intellect rather than a combination of heart and mind. The muscles at the back of the neck and shoulders (among other muscles) are overtaxed, which can lead to tension headaches.

To check your posture, stand with your feet hip-width apart and have a friend look at you from the side. If your bones are stacked one on top of another, they will hold your body upright with minimal effort: a vertical line through the center of your ear should intersect the centers of your shoulder joint, hip joint, and knee.

If you have head forward posture, restore alignment by gliding your chin in toward your throat until the ear and shoulder line up. If the hip joints are forward of the shoulders, slide the pelvis back under the shoulders. This correction may make you feel as if you are leaning forward like a gorilla, but it's a step in the right direction.

Once your ear, shoulder, hip, and knee are in alignment, check that your breathing is still relaxed and your spine has its natural curves. In a healthy spine, there is a gentle inward curve in the lower back, a gentle outward curve in the back of the chest, and another gentle inward curve in the neck. This is what yogis call a straight spine.

Now check the distribution of weight on your feet. Sway your body left and right, shifting your weight more onto one foot, then more onto the other, until you find a point in the center where equal weight is on both feet.

Now sway your body forward and backward, feeling your weight shift back and forth between the balls of your feet and your heels, until you come to a point in the middle where you feel the most balanced, most relaxed, and lightest in body, breath, and mind. Make sure your ear, shoulder, hip, and knee are still aligned. (figure 2) Breathe. Relax.

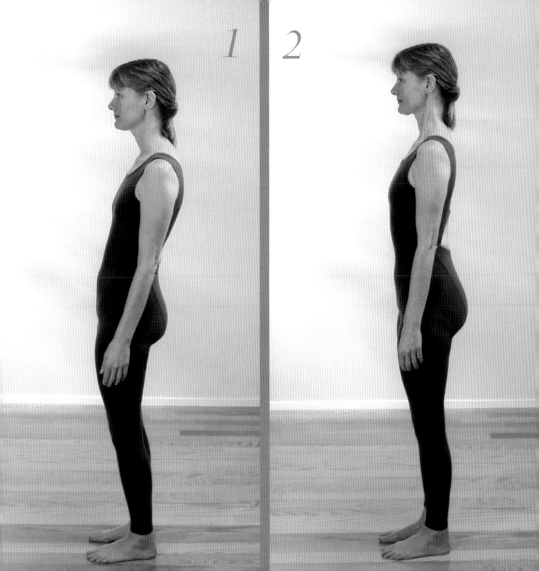

Finally, press your feet into the floor and lengthen your entire body upward, relaxing open through your abdomen and rib cage (front, sides, and back). Contrast how this feels with how you feel when your weight is collapsing down onto your legs and feet. If your weight is balanced and your posture straight, this position will feel exhilarating and effortless.

If you practice even these few basic aspects of posture, you will be well on your way to fewer tension headaches. Simply make one change at time, moving in a healthier direction rather than trying to perfect all aspects at once. After you have practiced for a while, your improved posture will feel natural to you.

Diaphragmatic Breathing

Many people breathe only with the chest, taking shallow breaths that deprive them of adequate oxygen and contribute directly to stress and anxiety. Breathing with the diaphragm has just the opposite affect: it both relaxes you and enables your lungs to absorb more oxygen.

The diaphragm is a dome-shaped muscle beneath your lungs. Its downward movement during inhalation causes air to flow into the lungs.

Although the diaphragm does move in shallow chest breathing, it plays a greater role in full diaphragmatic breathing, where it gently pushes your abdominal organs outward as you inhale.

Diaphragmatic breathing is easiest if you lie on your back on the floor. Try it: let your entire body relax, close your eyes, and rest one hand over your navel. Breathe easily, without forcing your breath to be either deep or shallow. Notice how your abdomen lifts your hand with each inhalation and relaxes down with each exhalation. This is how you breathe when you are relaxed.

This same abdominal action should take place when you are sitting or standing. However, due to poor posture habits—and perhaps the desire to look thin—many people hold their abdomens in and breathe only with the chest. It takes awareness and practice to keep the abdominal muscles relaxed, but it's much healthier to breathe that way.

Throughout the yoga exercises below, unless otherwise instructed, breathe diaphragmatically through the nose. It will reduce stress, relax your body and mind, nourish your cells, and increase the effectiveness of the exercises. In just a week or two you can form new breathing habits that will feel as natural as the old ones, but will provide far more health benefits for the rest of your life.

To deepen your relaxation and help you focus your mind, breathe slowly during these routines—as slowly as you can without discomfort.

Full Yogic Breath

A diaphragmatic inhalation is the first phase of the Full Yogic Breath, also known as the three-part breath. As you continue to inhale after the abdomen expands, the lower ribs will expand to the sides, creating the second phase of the Full Yogic Breath. The third phase completes the inhalation as the chest expands and the lungs completely fill with air.

The full yogic exhalation immediately follows; there is no holding of the breath beyond what happens naturally. The exhalation also comes in three parts: first the chest relaxes into normal position, then the ribs come back in, and finally the abdomen returns to its initial position. Exhalation should be the same duration as inhalation.

Full Yogic Breaths should create no strain, no sense of filling the lungs to absolute capacity. The breaths should be slow and easeful, with each inhalation and exhalation lasting about 5 seconds, more or less according to comfort.

The three phases of inhalation and exhalation should flow one into the other rather than be rigid or separated. Think of the inhalation as a gradual upward expansion of the torso, and the exhalation as a downward relaxation. The Full Yogic Breath alone, when performed slowly and with deep concentration, can often be an effective headache remedy.

Main Routine

The instructions for exercises 1–8 below assume a standing position. If you adapt them to sitting on a chair, sit upright with a straight spine, away from the back of the chair. If your knees are much lower than your hips when sitting on the chair, place a cushion under your feet.

The exercises in this routine are safe for most people. Nevertheless, you should do only what feels comfortable. Never push to the point of pain or discomfort. Be extra careful if you have had problems with shoulder or spinal injuries or weakness.

Once you have learned these exercises, the routine takes less than 20 minutes. For even better results, hold the poses for a longer period of time than suggested here, provided you are comfortable doing so.

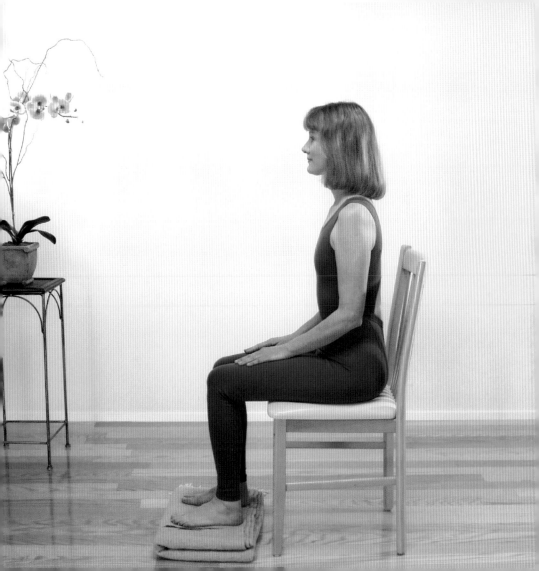

1. Practice Correct Standing Posture: Mountain Pose

Find your correct standing posture and practice staying relaxed in it for at least 30 seconds. Let the breath flow easily, with your chest open and abdomen soft. This is itself a yoga posture: Mountain Pose. (see right)

2. Full Yogic Breath

In the Mountain Pose, take 3–6 slow Full Yogic Breaths, growing a bit taller with each inhalation, and more relaxed without losing your height with each exhalation.

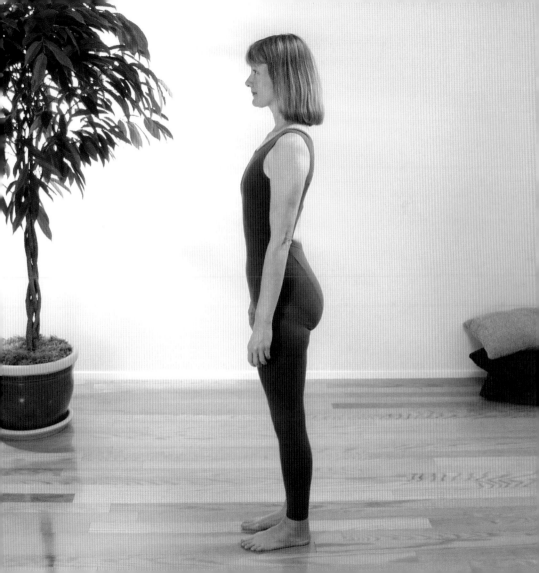

3. Standing Cat Stretch

Bend at the hips, keeping your spine straight, and place your palms on your thighs just above your knees. (figure a)

Inhale; then as you exhale, tuck your pelvis under and slowly round your spine, one vertebra at a time, from the base to the top of the spine, like a cat arching its back. Finish the exhalation by tucking your chin to your chest. (figure b)

As you slowly inhale, tip the pelvis forward as though your sit-bones were rotating backward and up, arching your spine in the opposite way, one vertebra at a time, from the base to the top of the spine. (Your sit-bones are the bony protuberances on the bottom of your pelvis which complain when you sit too long on a hard surface.) Finish the inhalation by lengthening through your neck and reaching for the sky through the crown of your head. (figure c) Avoid bending the neck backward sharply.

Slowly exhale and once again round your spine from the bottom upward. Continue for 4 more breaths. On your last inhalation, return to Mountain Pose.

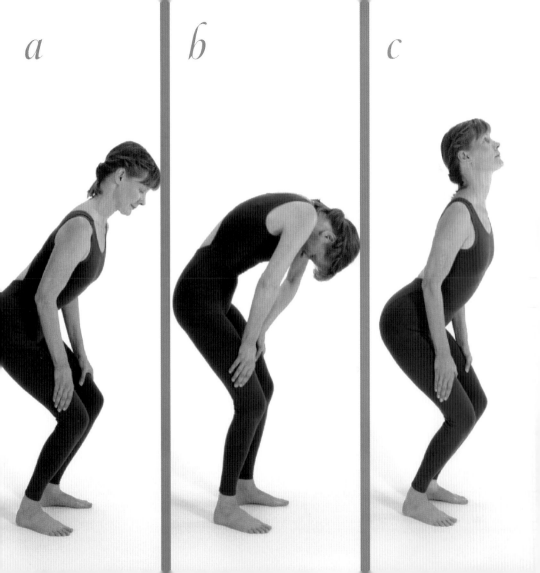

a *b* *c*

4. Circle of Joy

Place your palms together at your heart.

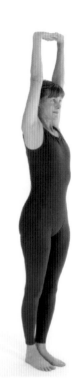

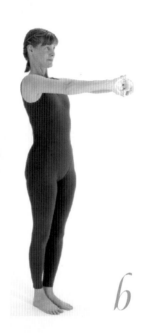

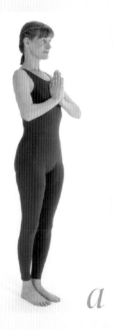

a

b

c

Inhaling, interlace your fingers. As you exhale, press your palms forward and outward at shoulder level, stretching through your shoulders.

Inhaling, circle your hands upward, extending through your palms and lengthening your spine.

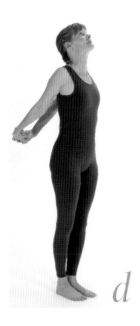

d

As you exhale, release your hands and circle them down behind you, interlacing your fingers once again. Inhale as you lengthen backward and upward through the arms and hands, forward and upward through the breastbone.

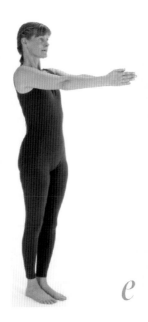

e

As you exhale, release your hands and circle them back in front, stretching forward through the fingertips.

Inhaling, bring your palms back together in the starting position at the heart and interlace the fingers. This completes one cycle. Do a total of 4 cycles, resting briefly after the last cycle.

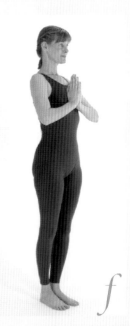

f

77

5. Eagle Arms

Bring your left arm up in front of you and bend it at the elbow, with your upper arm horizontal, and forearm vertical in front of your nose. Wrap your right arm underneath and around the left, until the palms come together.

Keeping your chest lifted and open, raise and lower your elbows until you find the position that affords the best stretch of your shoulders and upper back. As you hold the position and breathe easily, feel the release of tension throughout your upper body: shoulders, upper back, arms, and wrists. With each exhalation, visualize the released energy pouring into your spine, your center.

Affirm mentally:

At the center of life's storms
I stand serene.

Hold this position for at least 30 seconds, continuing the affirmation. Repeat on the other side, with left arm wrapping underneath right, for the same amount of time.

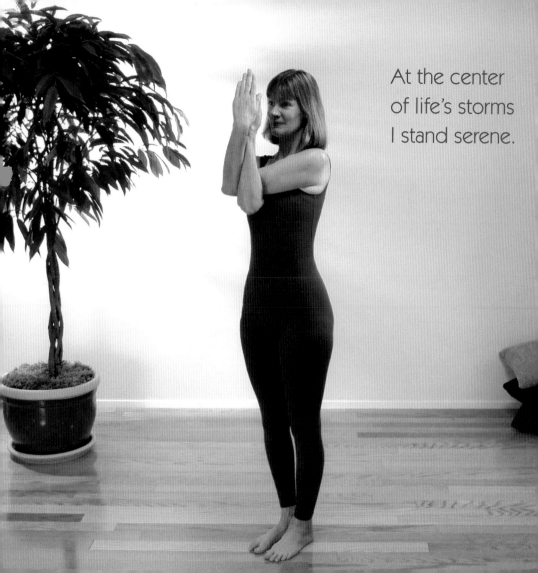

At the center
of life's storms
I stand serene.

Variation

If you cannot bring your palms together (this is quite common), drape a yoga strap between your left thumb and forefinger. After wrapping your right arm as far as it will go around the left, grasp the strap with both hands and as your shoulders relax, gradually work your hands closer together.

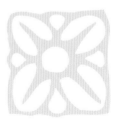

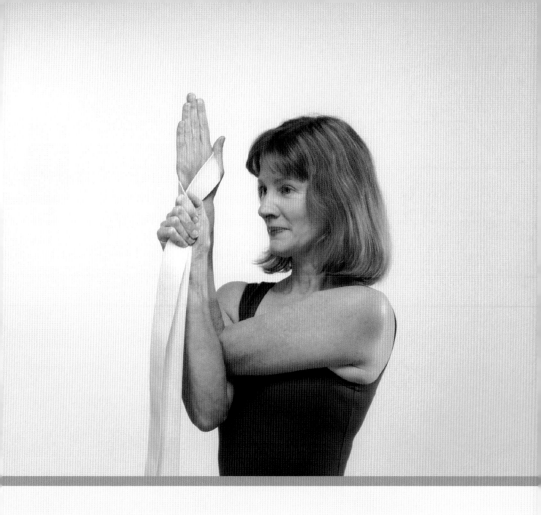

At the center of life's storms I stand serene.

6. Hold Elbows Overhead

Inhaling, circle your arms out to the sides and up over your head. Exhale and bend your elbows, grasping the opposite elbow with each hand. Relax your shoulders.

Breathing normally, lengthen up through the elbows with each inhalation. With each exhalation, relax the elbows backward behind you slightly. Do this for 30 seconds.

Caution

If your shoulders are tight, take care that you do not become sway-backed in this exercise. You may need to interlace your fingers with bent elbows rather than holding opposite elbows.

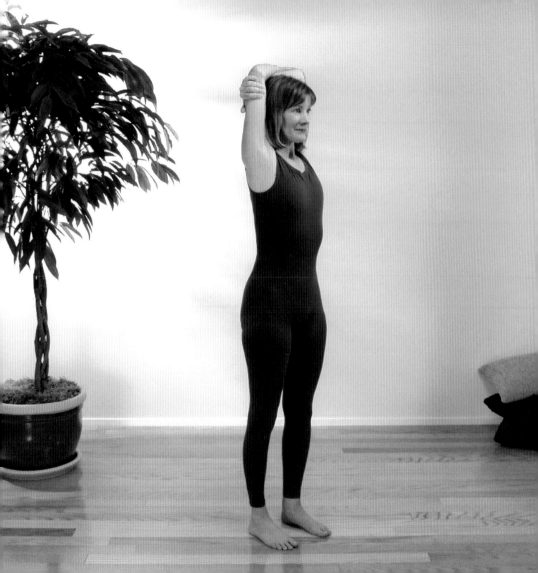

7. Neck Rechargers

These five exercises call for tensing and relaxing various muscles in your neck. When you tense, do so in smooth progression, from low to medium to high tension, so high that the muscles vibrate with energy. Similarly, relax smoothly from high to medium to low to no tension. Each set of tensing and relaxing should take about 3 seconds. Let your breath flow naturally while doing this; don't hold it.

Tense the front of your neck, then relax. Repeat 2 times.

Tense the left side of your neck, then relax. Tense the right side of your neck, then relax. Alternate sides, tensing and relaxing each side 2 more times.

Relax your chin to your chest (figure a). As you slowly inhale, draw your head upright and slightly back (figure b), tensing the muscles of the back of your neck as though some force were trying to keep your head down. As you exhale, slowly relax your chin back to your chest. Repeat 2 more times.

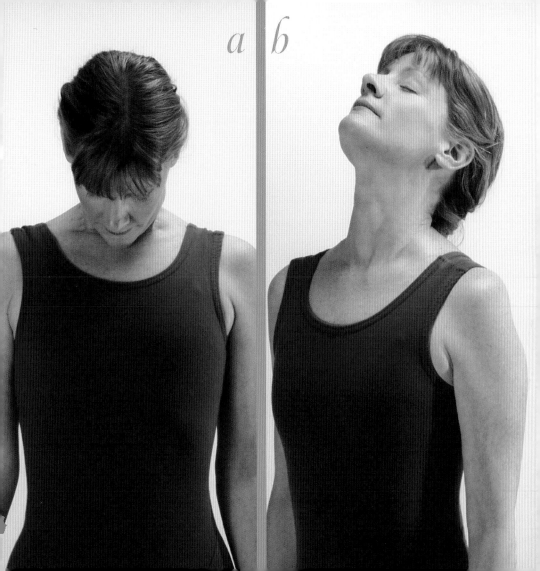

a *b*

Next, with moderate tension throughout all the neck muscles, make small circles with your head and neck three times in one direction, then three times in the opposite direction. (see right, figures a–d)

Finally, without any tension, circle your head three times in one direction, then three times in the opposite direction. Keep a sense of length in your neck; do not let your head roll around like a rag doll.

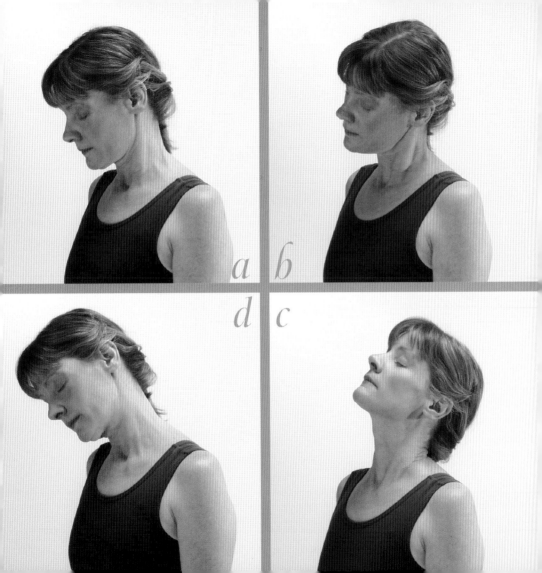

a *b*

d *c*

Variation

If you feel discomfort in your neck during the last movement, make the circles smaller and lift your shoulders to cradle your neck. (see a-d at right)

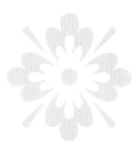

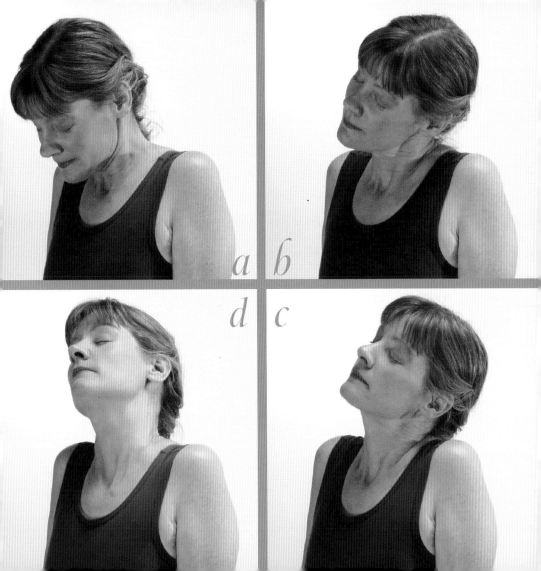

a *b*

d *c*

8. 6-Way Neck Stretches

As you do the following exercises, keep your torso upright, chest open. The only part of your spine that bends is the neck.

a. Interlace your fingers behind your head. Inhale and lengthen your neck, then exhale and bring your chin to your chest. (figure left)

Don't force your head down; simply let the weight of your hands and arms gently stretch the back of your neck. Stay in this position for another breath, then inhale and straighten up, exhale and bring your head forward and to your left, chin over left breast pocket. (figure right)

Stay in this position for another breath, gently stretching the back right part of your neck. Then inhale and straighten up, exhale and bring your head forward and to your right, stretching the back left part of your neck. Stay there for another breath, then inhale and straighten to the starting position. Repeat this sequence 4 more times.

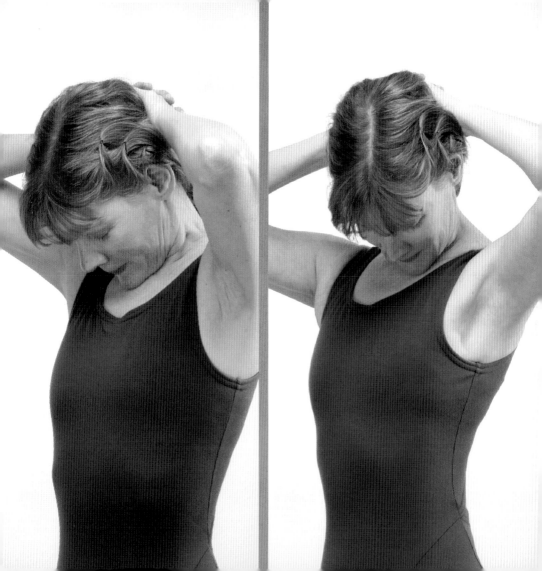

b. Place the first three fingers of both hands in the small indentation just below the base of your skull. Inhale and draw your head back, using your fingers to lift the skull and lengthen the neck until you feel a stretch in the front of your neck. (figure 1)

Exhale as you return to the starting position. Repeat 4 more times, then relax your hands to your sides.

c. Inhale and lengthen your neck. Exhale and rotate your head to the left as far as is comfortable. (figure 2)

Pause there for a moment, then inhale and rotate back to center. Exhale and rotate your head to the right as far as comfortable. Continue, going to each side 4 more times.

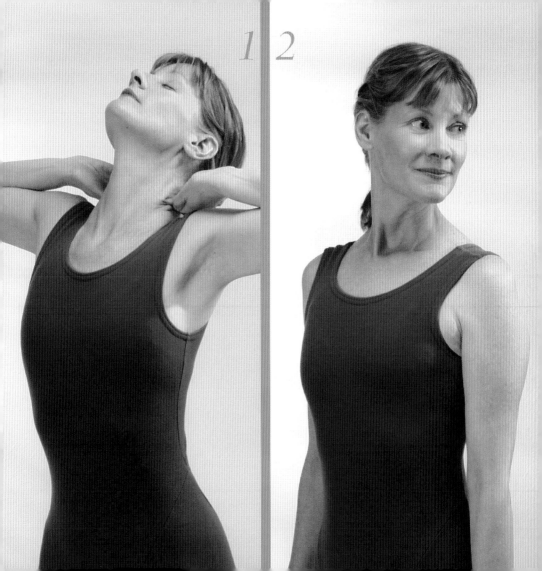

d. Bring your right arm behind your back and bend it at the elbow. Bring your left arm over the top of your head and left hand just above the right ear. Inhale and lengthen your neck, then exhale and gently use your left arm to draw the left ear toward the left shoulder. Keep your shoulder relaxed and spine vertical; do not lean your body to the left. (figure left)

Do not force the stretch. Let the weight of your hand and arm stretch the right side of your neck. Stay in this position for another breath, then inhale and straighten up. Repeat 4 more times. Then do the exercise to the other side.

e. Inhaling, slowly glide your chin horizontally forward as far as is comfortable without moving your torso forward. (figure center)

Exhale and draw the chin back in toward the throat as far as is comfortable without moving your torso backward. Repeat 4 more times. (figure right)

f. Imagining that the tip of your nose is a pencil, draw a figure eight in the air in front of you, 5 times. Make the figure eights as large as possible. Then draw figure eights in the opposite direction, 5 times. Next, draw sideways figure eights, 5 times, again making them as large as possible. Repeat in the opposite direction, 5 times.

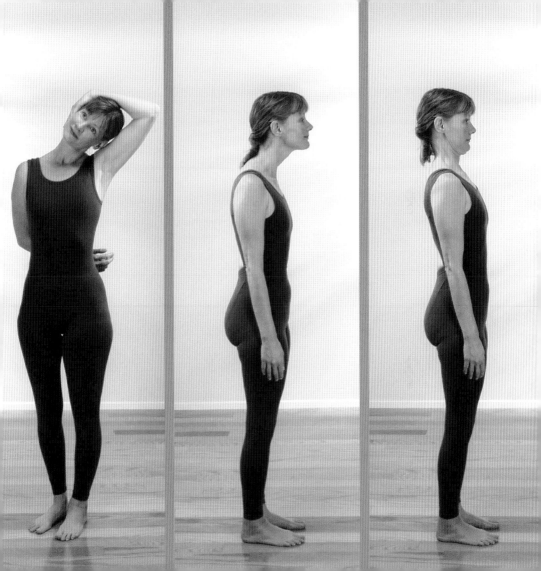

9. Hare Pose

Come down onto your knees, then sit back onto your heels with your thighs parallel. Bend forward from the hips to lower your abdomen onto your thighs and forehead onto the floor. From this initial position, reach behind and grasp your heels, curling your fingers inward toward opposite hands. (figure 1)

Bring your forehead as close to your knees as is comfortable, and place the crown of your head on the floor. Continue holding your heels as you inhale and lift your buttocks, stretching your arms straight. Rest only a small amount of your weight on the crown of your head; most of your weight should be on your legs. (figure 2)

Relax your arms, shoulders, and upper back as you keep lifting through the legs to stretch and open the upper body. This pose helps you gain control over the energy in the spine, especially when you focus on stretching forward through the spine even as the hands resist forward movement. Hold the pose for 30 to 60 seconds, your breath smooth and natural, and affirm mentally:

> I am master of my energy.
> I am master of myself.

To exit, lower your buttocks back down to your heels, let go of your heels, and slowly settle back down to rest in the initial position.

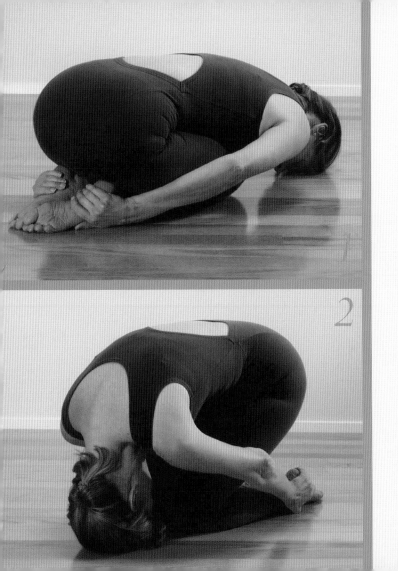

I am master

of my energy.

I am master

of myself.

If you cannot grasp your heels, you may be able to do so if you come up on your toes, or, loop a yoga strap around your heels and hold the strap with your hands. (figure 1)

If your neck is not strong, from the initial position bring your elbows to the floor alongside your eyes, palms on the floor. Inhale and lift your buttocks, rolling onto the crown of your head with the weight of your upper body carried on your forearms and elbows. From this position, roll forward gently to stretch the back of your neck. (figure 2)

Although this variation does not stretch the back and shoulders, it does give the benefits of inversion and a neck stretch.

If your knees are uncomfortable in the initial position, you can also do the Hare Pose on a chair: bend forward to rest your torso on your thighs. Reach back and grasp the chair's rear legs, then stretch forward to achieve a "dynamic resistance" effect similar to that of grasping the heels in the standard Hare Pose. (figure 3)

Cautions

Avoid turning your head to either side while in this pose. Pregnant women who are beyond their first trimester should avoid this pose, as should individuals with cardiovascular problems such as high blood pressure, cardiovascular disease, history of stroke, recent spinal injuries, or diseases or inflammations of the eyes, ears, or sinuses.

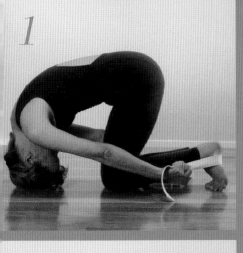

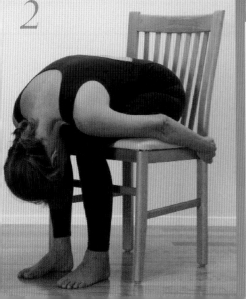

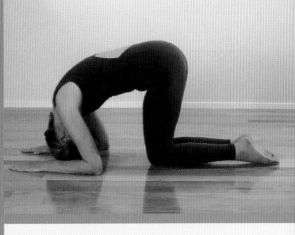

I am master

of my energy.

I am master

of myself.

10. Front-Stretching Pose

Return to an upright position, sitting back on your heels with thighs parallel. From this initial position, lean back and place your palms on the floor 12 to 18 inches behind you, fingers pointing backward. Tuck your pelvis. As you inhale, lift the buttocks off the heels and arch your body—from your knees all the way up through your neck—into a uniform backward bend. Lift and open the entire front of your body, especially your chest and shoulders, as you keep the pelvis tucked.

Transform this physical opening into an enthusiastic opening to life itself as you rise above worries and fears. Breathe in a smooth and natural rhythm, affirming silently:

> With a burst of energy,
> I rise to greet the world!

Hold this pose for 15–30 seconds. To exit, inhale and lengthen your spine, then exhale as you lower the buttocks back down onto the heels.

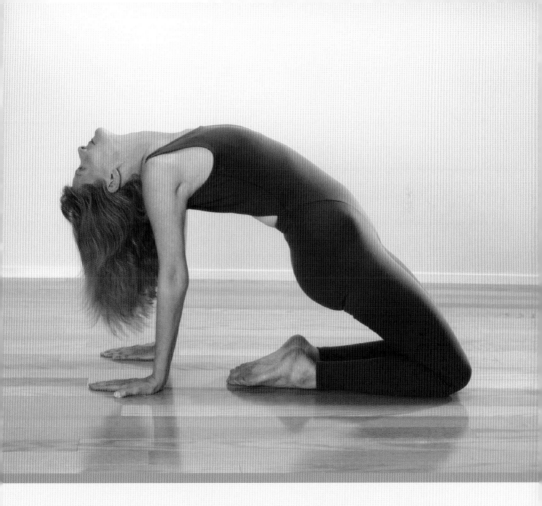

With a burst of energy, I rise to greet the world!

Variations

If your ankles are uncomfortable in the initial position, place a rolled towel under the fronts of your ankles. If your knees are uncomfortable in this position, place a cushion between the backs of your ankles and your buttocks. (figure 1)

If your knees are still uncomfortable, do this pose on a chair, leaving your buttocks down on the chair seat. (figure 2)

Cautions

Those with cardiovascular problems such as high blood pressure, cardiovascular disease, history of stroke, or recent spinal injuries should do only a gentle version of this pose. For those with vulnerable knees, it's usually best to do this pose on a chair.

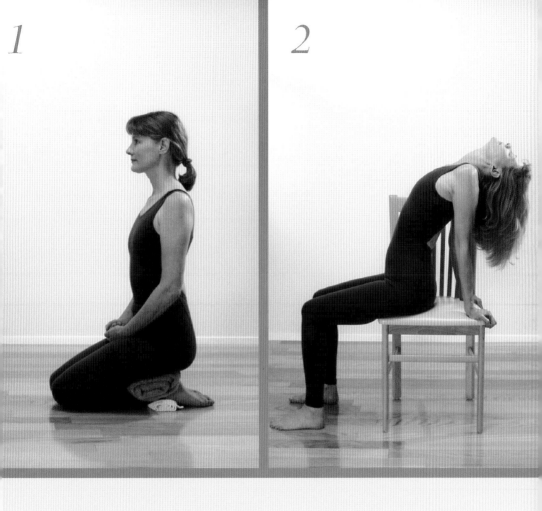

With a burst of energy, I rise to greet the world!

11. Child Pose

Relax your arms at your sides and bend forward from the hips, leading with your chest and keeping your spine long as you lay your abdomen over your thighs and rest your forehead on the floor, palms facing up by your feet.

Relax your whole body, especially your arms and legs, which were so active in the last two poses. Breathe in a smooth, natural flow, letting your breathing massage and open your back and shoulders.

Affirm in your mind,

I relax from outer involvement into my inner haven of peace.

Remain in this pose for 30 seconds.

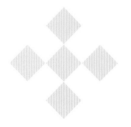

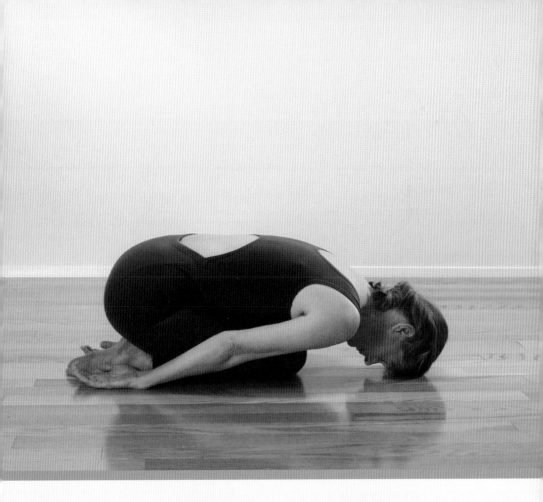

I relax from outer involvement into my
inner haven of peace.

If your ankles or knees are uncomfortable, use a rolled towel under the fronts of your ankles or a cushion between the backs of your ankles and your buttocks, as described above under variations for the Front-Stretching Pose. Also, you may find it more comfortable to bring your arms up beside your head and rest your head on one forearm. (see right)

Pregnant women and overweight persons should move their knees apart in this pose to prevent abdominal compression.

If you were using a chair for the Front-Stretching Pose, remain in the chair for the Child Pose and simply bend forward, resting your torso on your thighs, relaxing your neck completely, and letting your arms hang loosely to the floor.

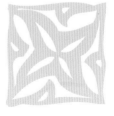

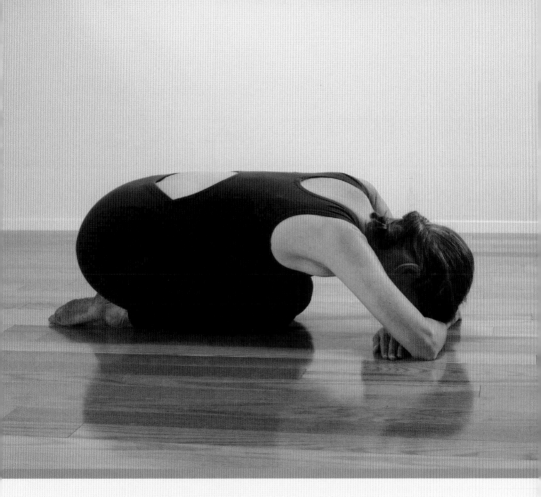

I relax from outer involvement into my
inner haven of peace.

12. Bridge Pose

Place a folded blanket on the floor and lie on your back on the blanket, with the tops of your shoulders 2 to 3 inches below the folded edge of the blanket, arms directly alongside your body on the blanket. Bend your knees and slide your feet in, about 4 to 6 inches from your buttocks and hip-width apart. Your feet should be parallel to each other. (figure 1)

Firmly tuck your pelvis, and on an inhalation, press the balls of your feet into the floor and slowly peel your spine off the floor, one vertebra at a time. Do not allow your knees to open wider than hip width.

Interlace your fingers behind your back, palms together, and roll your shoulders under, one side at a time, opening the front of your chest without closing off the back. Come up only as far as is comfortable. Keep your thighs parallel. Your shins should be vertical when you are in this pose (ask a friend to check); if not, slide your feet closer to or farther away from your head. (figure 2)

Once again you are opening the front of the body, this time as though offering yourself—body, mind, heart, and soul—upward to receive divine healing light. Breathe in a smooth and natural rhythm as you hold the pose for at least 30 seconds, mentally affirming,

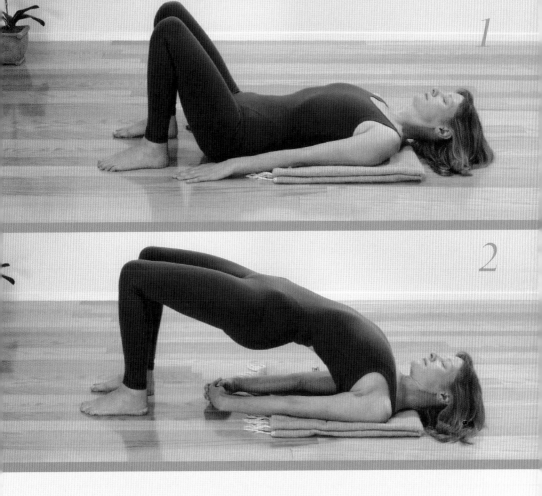

1

2

I offer every thought as a bridge to divine grace.

I offer every thought as a
bridge to divine grace.

To exit, exhale and lower your spine, vertebra by vertebra, back to the floor. Bring your knees up toward your chest, wrap your arms around them, and squeeze your thighs into your abdomen to release and stretch your lower back. Relax your legs to the floor, remove the blanket, and briefly lie resting on the floor.

Cautions

Avoid turning your head to either side while in this pose.

If you have a knee injury or vulnerability, use caution in this pose. It may relieve knee discomfort if you tie a yoga strap around your knees so they stay hip-width apart, then press actively into the confines of the strap during the pose. (see right)

If the discomfort persists, repeat the Front-Stretching Pose instead, concentrating this time on lifting the chest while drawing the chin strongly toward the chest to stretch the back of the neck.

Women who are menstruating or are pregnant beyond the first trimester should avoid this pose, as should individuals with cardiovascular problems such as high blood pressure, cardiovascular disease, history of stroke, recent spinal injuries, or diseases or inflammations of the eyes, ears, or sinuses. Instead, repeat the Front-Stretching Pose (see preceding paragraph).

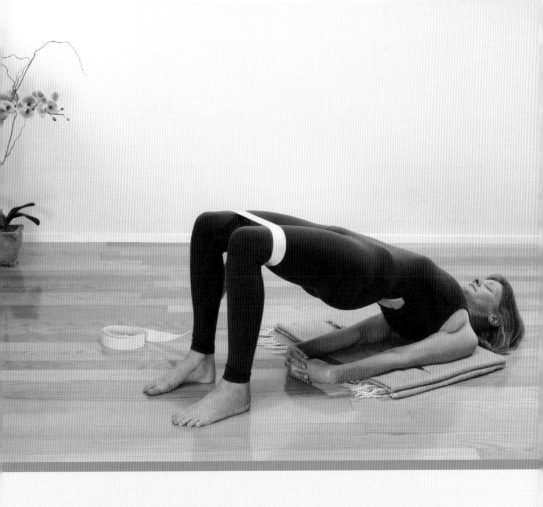

I offer every thought as a bridge to divine grace.

13. Fish Pose

Lie on your back, hands beneath your buttocks, arms straight and palms down. On an inhalation, firmly press your sit-bones into your hands and elbows into the floor, slowly drawing your body up into a backward bend. Keep your head in contact with the floor, sliding it closer to your body as you come up, but not so close that your neck bends sharply. Place only as much weight on your head as if you were standing upright resting a hand on your head.

Maintain a dynamic backward bend of your spine by lengthening actively through your legs, and pressing your elbows into the floor and sit-bones into the backs of your hands, while keeping your shoulder blades spread wide. Open your entire torso and the front of your neck.

This asana brings a feeling of expansiveness to the opening begun in the Bridge Pose. Visualize your awareness spreading in all directions like ripples from a stone dropped into a pond. Breathe naturally as you hold the pose for 30 seconds, affirming silently,

My soul floats on waves of cosmic light.

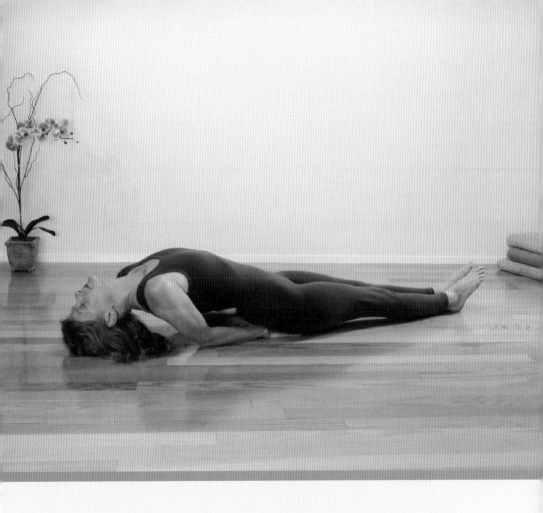

My soul floats on waves of cosmic light.

To exit, as you inhale press your elbows into the floor and bring your chin to your chest, lengthening the back of your neck. Then exhale and slowly lower yourself back to the floor, starting with your lumbar spine and finishing with your head. Lie resting for a moment to integrate the effects of the pose.

Cautions

If your wrists are uncomfortable, make sure they are not bent at a sideways angle. Your middle finger should align with your forearm.

Pregnant women who are beyond their first trimester should avoid this pose, as should individuals with cardiovascular problems such as high blood pressure, cardiovascular disease, history of stroke, recent spinal injuries, or diseases or inflammations of the eyes, ears, or sinuses. These persons can instead sit on the floor and rest the back of the head on a padded chair, opening the front of the neck without bending the neck backward sharply.

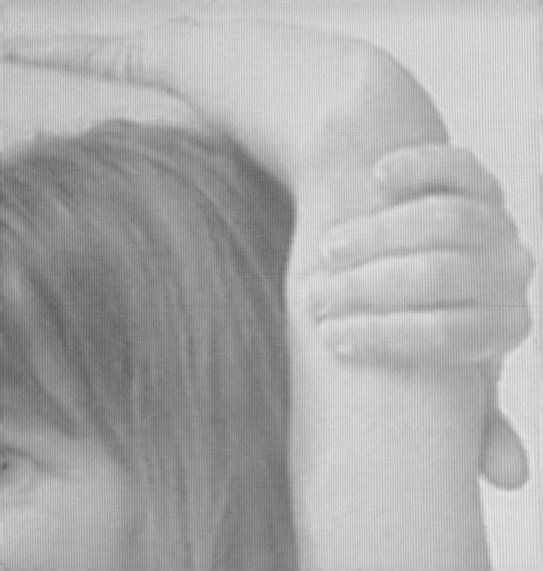

14. Supine Twist

Lying on your back, stretch your arms out to your sides, palms up. Bend your knees, slide your feet toward your buttocks, and shift your hips 4 to 6 inches to the left. Inhale, lift your feet, and bring your thighs to a vertical position, knees together; then exhale and roll your lower body to the right, releasing both knees toward the floor. Keep your left shoulder on the floor and both knees together; avoid letting your upper knee slide behind the lower knee. Let your right foot come to the floor so your legs can relax. Lift your head slightly and rotate your gaze out over your outstretched left arm, then lower your head to the floor in this rotated position.

This pose stretches and relaxes the muscles along the physical spine, helping to open the "energy spine," which is the central channel of life-force in the body. Breathe naturally as you hold the pose for 30 to 60 seconds, concentrating on letting go of tension and opening up the current of prana in your spine. Affirm in your mind,

I open to the flow of God's life within me.

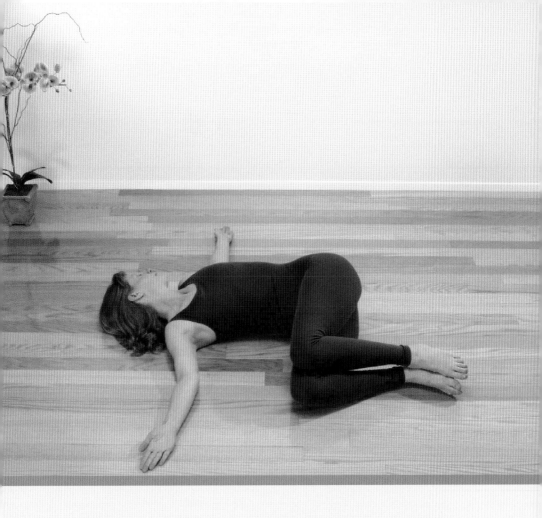

I open to the flow of God's life within me.

To exit, rotate your head back to center, inhale, and lengthen your spine, then as you exhale, roll your lower body back to center once again. Release both feet to the floor, slide your hips back to center, and rest briefly before repeating to the other side.

Variations

If your lower back is uncomfortable, bring your knees closer to your face.

Pregnant women and overweight persons can bend the knees less to avoid abdominal compression.

Caution

Individuals with recent spinal injuries should avoid this pose.

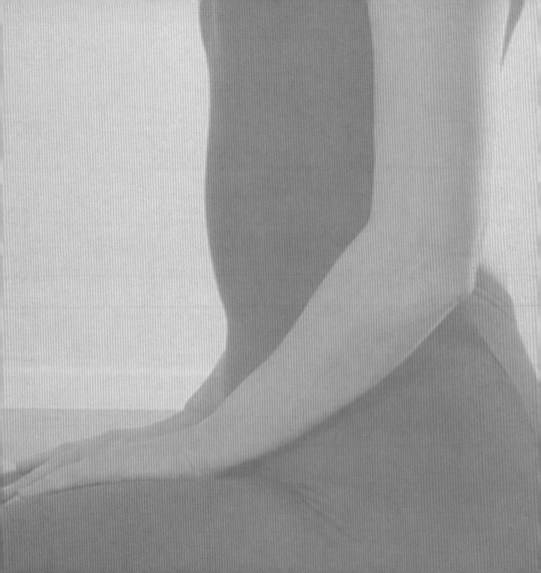

15. Deep Relaxation in the Corpse Pose

Lie on your back and stretch your legs away from your head to lengthen your spine. Rest your feet a little wider than hip-width apart, and let them roll out to the sides. Stretch your shoulders down away from your ears. Move your shoulder blades down your back, keeping them wide apart. Open your inner arms and palms toward the sky, with your hands far enough away from your body to maintain an open feeling in your armpits, but not so far away that your shoulders feel restricted. Lift your head and look down your body to check that all body parts are sym-metrically arranged. Inhale and extend through the back of your neck, then exhale as you lay your head back down. (see right)

Now you are prepared to experience deep relaxation. This is one of the most important poses for any headache sufferer, for both prevention and intervention, because it promotes a deep feeling of peaceful release. Let your breath be smooth and natural, not controlling it at all. Especially with each exhalation, concentrate on releasing and relaxing. Affirm mentally,

Bones, muscles, movement I surrender now; anxiety, elation and depression, churning thoughts—all these I give into the hands of peace.

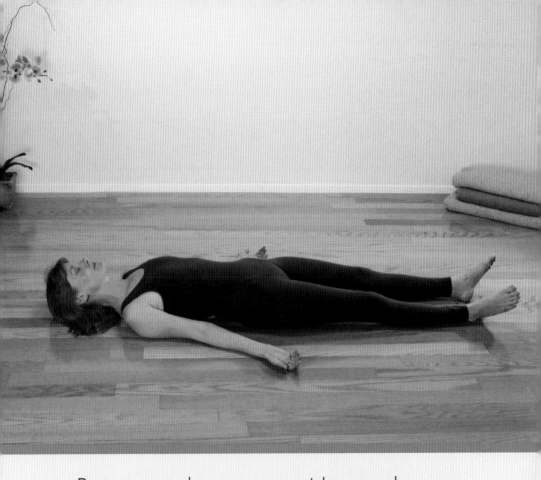

Bones, muscles, movement I surrender now;
anxiety, elation and depression, churning thoughts
—all these I give into the hands of peace.

Notice how this affirmation speaks to every level of your being: physical (bones, muscles, movement), emotional (anxiety, elation, depression), mental (thoughts), and spiritual (peace). Enjoy the freedom that comes from letting go on every level. Stay in this position for at least 5 minutes, moving gradually from repetition of the affirmation into a deep, wordless absorption in peace.

To return to a sitting position, slowly bring your knees to your chest and roll over onto your right side. Pause for a few breaths, then slowly come upright by pressing into the floor with your left hand and right elbow. Let your head be the last body part to come up. Sit in silence for a minute or so before getting up to move with grace and peacefulness into the next activity of your day.

Variations

If you like, place a cloth over your eyes during this pose to help you go inward.

If your lower back feels compressed in this pose, place a cushion or a rolled blanket under your knees. If your cervical spine feels compressed or needs support, place a small cushion or a rolled towel under your neck. (see right)

If you have large shoulders that cause your chin to point up in the air when you lie down, place a cushion or folded blanket under your head.

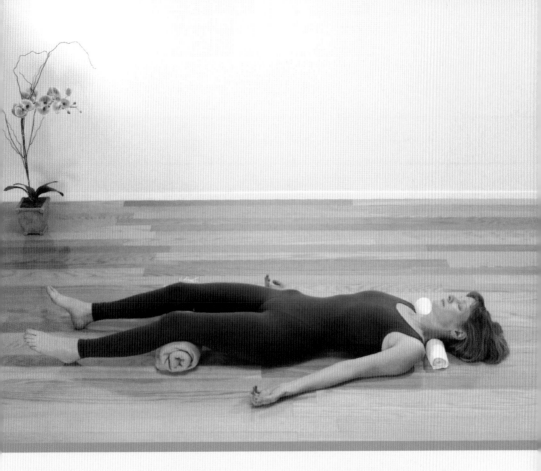

Bones, muscles, movement I surrender now;
anxiety, elation and depression, churning thoughts
—all these I give into the hands of peace.

Caution

Pregnant women should do this pose lying on the left side with cushions under the head, between the knees, under the abdomen, and anywhere else where support will enhance comfort.

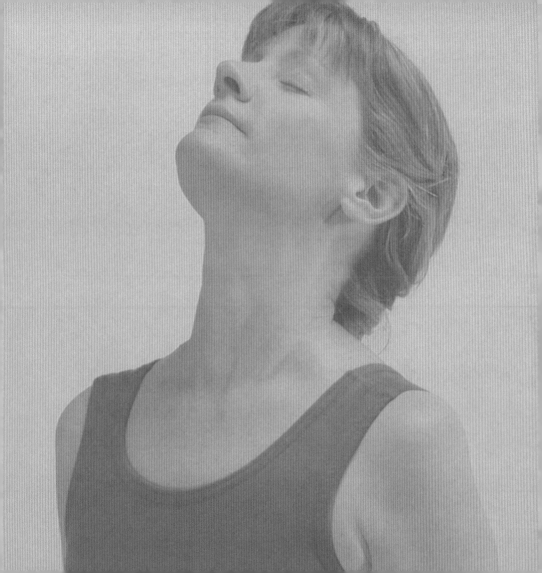

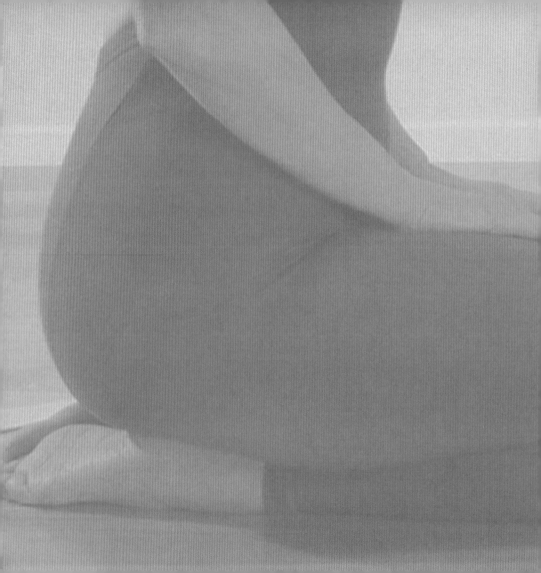

Chapter Seven

Additional Postures

When you feel comfortable doing the postures in the Main Routine—and ready to find a deeper level of relaxation—try the following (see Chapter Ten for sequencing):

Optional:

More Time in

the Mountain Pose

At the beginning of the routine, spend 1 to 2 minutes in Mountain Pose, consciously practicing correct standing posture and the Full Yogic Breath. Cultivate an attitude of relaxed alertness, mentally affirming,

I am calm,

with each inhalation, and

I am poised,

with each exhalation. Repeat after doing the 6-Way Neck Stretches.

Optional:

Ear-Closing Pose

This is one of the most effective yoga postures for reducing neck and shoulder tension. Practice it immediately after the Bridge Pose, in which case use two blankets for the Bridge Pose.

Still lying on the blankets, bring your arms to your sides, palms down. Bend your knees and slide your feet toward your buttocks. Inhale and draw your thighs toward your chest, then exhale and push your hands and the backs of your arms into the floor, bringing your buttocks off the floor and your legs back over your head. Let your knees soften toward the floor past the sides of your head. If possible, lower your feet to the floor, with the tops of the feet resting on the floor. Bring your palms together and interlace your fingers, then roll your shoulders under to straighten your spine.

Maintain length in your spine as you slowly release your knees toward the floor. The spine may round somewhat; that's fine provided it feels comfortable. When you have reached your final position, relax

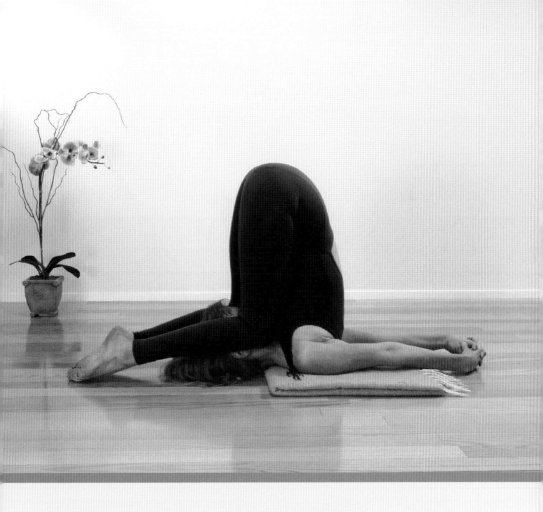

My boat of life floats lightly on tides of peace.

there, breathing smoothly and naturally. Because this pose offers a deep stretch of the neck, shoulders, and upper back, it is good to hold it as long as is comfortable and enjoyable—one minute or longer.

This asana is very restful for the brain, promoting a feeling of profound lightness and peace. Immerse yourself in that feeling by affirming mentally,

My boat of life floats lightly
on tides of peace.

To exit, inhale and press the backs of your shoulders into the floor to lift your legs slightly, then exhale and slowly uncurl your spine back onto the floor, one vertebra at a time. Press the backs of your arms into the floor to control your descent.

Remove the blanket and lie still on your back for 30 seconds to integrate the effects of the pose.

Cautions

Every movement of this pose should be slow and graceful, not using momentum to throw your legs overhead. If momentum is the only way in which you can enter the pose, then you are not yet ready for the pose.

Women who are menstruating or are pregnant beyond the first trimester should avoid this pose, as should individuals with cardiovascular problems such as high blood pressure, cardiovascular disease, history of stroke, recent spinal injuries, or diseases or inflammations of the eyes, ears, or sinuses.

beginners. It is best to learn them in person from a qualified instructor; see the chapter "Additional Steps You Can Take with Ananda Yoga." Insert one or both of these poses into the Main Routine before or after the Ear-Closing Pose.

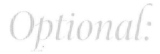

Optional:

Plow Pose and
Shoulderstand

While very effective for reducing neck and shoulder tension, these poses are not usually taught to

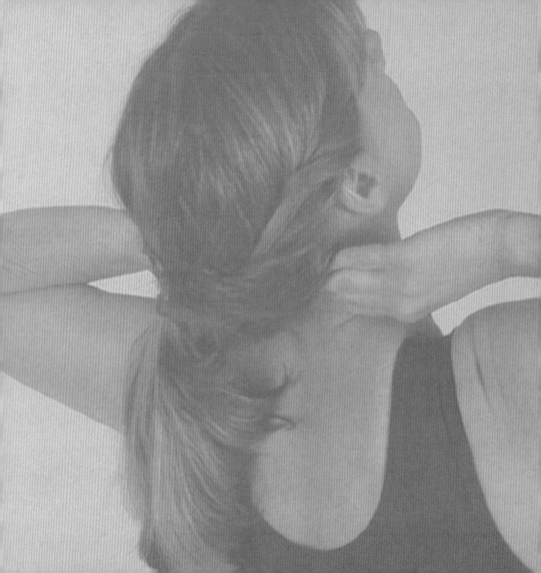

Chapter Eight

Ananda Yoga Headache Intervention Routine

When you have been unable to avoid a headache, try part or all of this Intervention Routine. Avoid any of the exercises that feel uncomfortable to you.

1. Full Yogic Breath

While standing, sitting, or lying on your back, take a number of slow, even, deep full yogic breaths. Avoid the strain of taking large inhalations; keep them full but comfortable, emphasizing relaxation on the exhalations.

2. The Basic Five
(Exercises 4–8 of the Main Routine)

If muscle tension has caused your headache, some of these exercises can be helpful if done very gently. However, if you have a migraine, you may prefer to skip them all.

3. Supported Extended Child Pose

Sit down on your heels in front of a chair that has a padded seat. Lean forward and rest your forehead and arms on the seat, elbows comfortably bent and palms down.

Hold the pose for as long as desired, breathing with ease. Mentally affirm,

I relax from outer involvement
into my inner haven of peace.

Come up very slowly and sit upright for at least a minute before getting up.

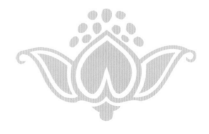

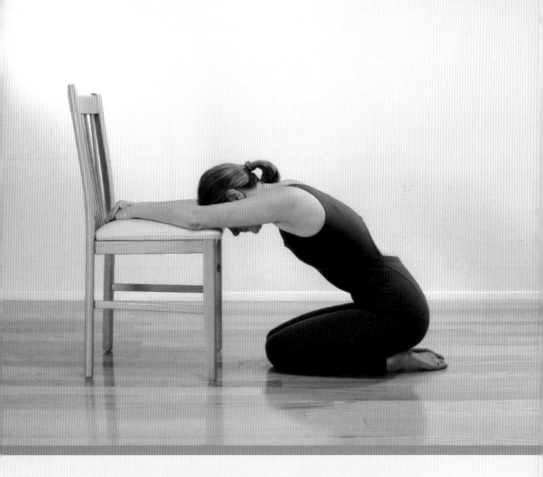

I relax from outer involvement into my
inner haven of peace.

If your ankles are uncomfortable in this position, place a rolled towel under the fronts of your ankles. If your knees are uncomfortable in this position, place a cushion between the backs of your ankles and your buttocks. (figure 1)

If you are still uncomfortable, you may prefer to sit in a chair instead, leaning forward to rest your forehead and arms on a cushion placed on top of a table. (figure 2)

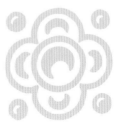

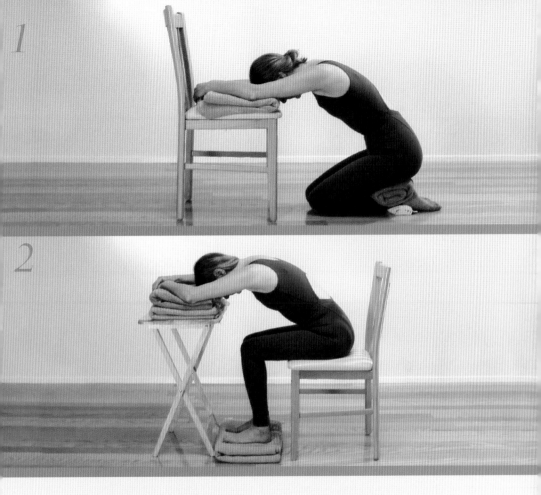

1

2

I relax from outer involvement into my
inner haven of peace.

4. Supported Corpse Pose

Lie down in the Corpse Pose, with a rolled blanket under the knees, a cushion or folded blanket under the head, a rolled towel under the neck, and a cloth over the eyes.

Breathe with natural ease, and find a place of stillness and peace within you, despite the headache. Relax away from discomfort, into that peace, as you mentally affirm,

Bones, muscles, movement I surrender now; anxiety, elation and depression, churning thoughts—all these I give into the hands of peace.

Stay in the pose for as long as desired. When finished, slowly bring your knees to your chest and roll over onto your right side. Pause, then slowly bring yourself upright by pressing into the floor with your left hand and right elbow. Let your head be the last body part to come up. Sit quietly for a minute or two before getting up.

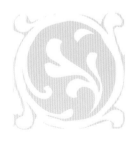

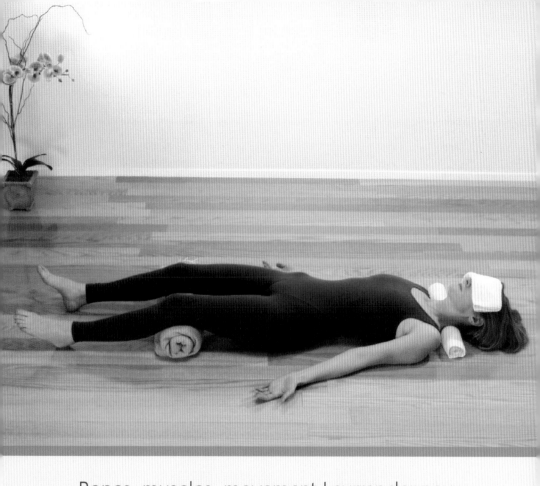

Bones, muscles, movement I surrender now;
anxiety, elation and depression, churning thoughts
—all these I give into the hands of peace.

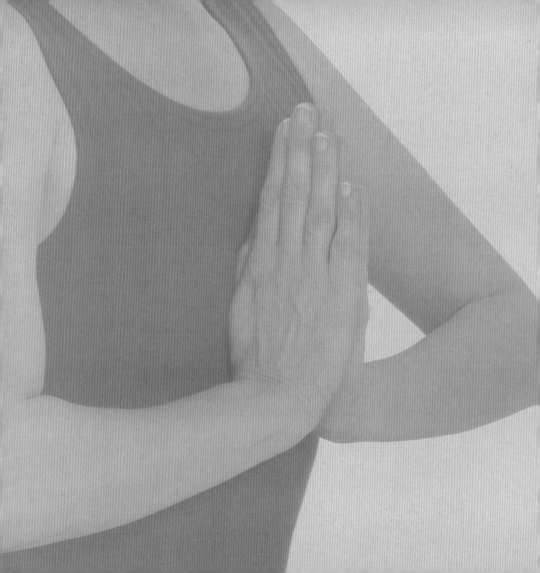

Chapter Nine

More You Can Do for Your Headaches

If you're a chronic headache sufferer, you'll want to explore every reasonable solution to get rid of your headaches for good. Here's an overview of some other medical recommendations that you may wish to use in addition to your Ananda Yoga exercises to ensure you get the maximum benefit from your program. You'll see that the recommendations are different for each type of headache.

More Help for Migraines

For migraine prevention probably the most effective and common sense approach is to avoid anything you know to be a migraine trigger for you, such as inadequate amounts of sleep or certain foods, like red wine. You'll want to keep a watchful eye on your emotional state and stress levels. Taking a "mental health day" away from your work to avoid a stress-induced migraine may make more sense than missing three days once a severe migraine takes hold. A regular exercise program of 30–45 minutes per day, about five times a week, can be an excellent stress management tool. Doing a more extensive program of Ananda Yoga, including both meditation and yoga postures, can also have a dramatically positive effect on your response to stress.

You may want to review any medications you're taking for any other medical problem, to be sure that your headaches aren't being caused as a side effect. Women who are postmenopausal and are taking hormones may find that their estrogen supplement increases their migraines.

For very mild migraine headaches, ibuprofen (like Advil), taken as early in the headache as possible, can prove effective. Studies have shown that acetaminophen (Tylenol) doesn't seem to work very well with migraines. Ibuprofen should not be taken on a daily basis for headaches because it can cause problems with "rebound headaches" and has its own side effect risks. Pain relievers that are combined with caffeine are more effective than those that do not include it. Some chronic sufferers have found that drinking a caffeinated beverage along with their pain reliever seems to boost its effectiveness.

If you are having migraines that are incapacitating, or are having headaches more than a few times a year, you may want to consult your physician concerning one of the new triptans like Imitrex, Zomig, Maxalt, Axert, or Amerge mentioned earlier, which can stop an attack cold. These are often effective, particularly if taken early in the migraine's progress. For those with frequent migraines, such as one a week, a prescription from your doctor for a preventive medication such as atenolol (a beta-blocker), valproate (an anti-seizure medication), or amitriptyline (a tricyclic antidepressant) may help.

Riboflavin, vitamin B2, has shown promise for migraine prevention in a small study and appears to decrease the frequency of migraines for many people. A dose of 400 mg a day is recommended and this can be purchased without a prescription and taken safely. There are some herbal treatments for migraine, such as feverfew, that have shown promise.

Recently, Botox (botulinum toxin) injections have proven helpful in some limited trials for those with difficult-to-treat migraines.

Biofeedback training can be used to teach you how to "short circuit" the onset of a migraine, but the effectiveness is about the same as the kind of relaxation training we have presented with Ananda Yoga. Acupuncture, homeopathy, chiropractic, hypnosis, and oxygen therapy have not conclusively shown that they alleviate migraines and it's best to consider them a last resort.

More on Tension Headaches

The treatment options for tension headaches are a little different than for migraines. The majority of mild tension headaches can be managed with acetaminophen (Tylenol) or ibuprofen in the standard doses noted on the bottle if they do not respond to simple relaxation measures like Ananda Yoga. Massage of the neck and scalp or hot/cold packs applied there can also help ease a tension headache. Chiropractic manipulations of the neck may also be helpful for tension headaches. Botox injections have recently been shown, in limited studies, to be effective in difficult-to-treat tension headaches.

A regular exercise program such as mentioned in the migraine headache section as well as a more extensive Ananda Yoga program would together be a good preventive regimen for tension headaches and helpful for general stress management.

If you have recurrent tension headaches, discuss the possibility of depression or anxiety problems with your doctor. Frequent headaches may be a symptom of underlying psychological distress.

Ananda Yoga Will Add to Any Medical Program

You can see that Ananda Yoga Therapy offers an easy, time-efficient way to help prevent both migraines and tension headaches. In addition, it will increase the efficacy of whatever other therapy, standard or alternative, your doctor recommends. You will have added to your lifestyle surprisingly powerful techniques that will give you a new sense of well-being and calm control far beyond the immediate goal of help for headaches.

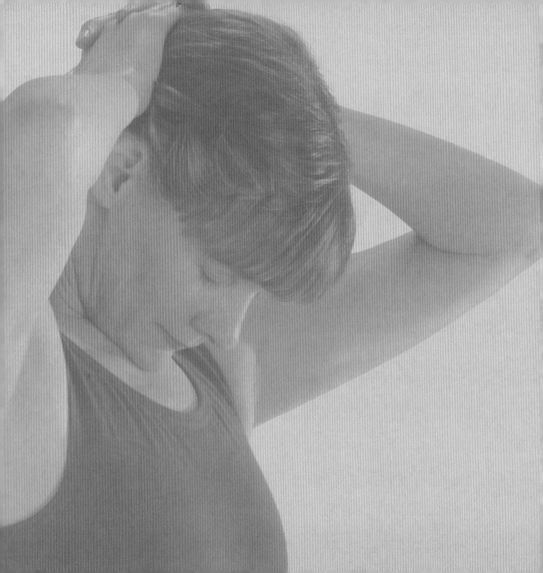

Chapter Ten

Summary of the Main Routine

The optional exercises may be inserted after you are completely comfortable with the Main Routine.

1. Mountain Pose
(30 seconds)

2. Full Yogic Breath
(3-6 breaths)

Optional: (1-2 minutes)

I am calm,
with each inhalation,
I am poised.
with each exhalation.

3. Standing Cat Stretch
(5 breaths)

4. Circle of Joy
(4 cycles)

5. Eagle Arms
(30 seconds each side)
At the center of life's storms
I stand serene.

6. Hold Elbows Overhead
(30 seconds)

7. Neck Rechargers

Front of neck

Alternate
left/right sides
of neck

Back of neck

Small circles
with head and
neck, tensing
throughout
neck

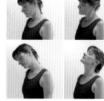

Small circles
without
tension

8. 6-Way Neck Stretches

a. Forward, forward-left, forward-right
(5 times)

b. Lift head up and back
(5 times)

c. Rotate neck left and right
(5 times each direction)

d. Draw ear toward shoulder
(5 times each side)

e. Glide chin forward and back (5 times)

f. Figure eights with the tip of the nose (vertical 5 times each direction, then horizontal 5 times each direction)

Optional: Mountain Pose

(1-2 minutes, using the Full Yogic Breath)
I am calm,
with each inhalation,
I am poised
with each exhalation.

9. Hare Pose

(30–60 seconds, then rest in Child Pose for 30 seconds)
I am master of my energy,
I am master of myself.

10. Front-Stretching Pose
(15–30 seconds)
With a burst of energy,
I rise to greet the world!

11. Child Pose
(30 seconds)
I relax from outer involvement
into my inner haven of peace.

12. Bridge Pose
(at least 30 seconds)
I offer every thought
as a bridge to divine grace.

Optional: Shoulderstand
(30–60 seconds)
God's peace now floods my being.

Optional: Plow Pose
(30–60 seconds)
New life, new consciousness now
flood my brain!

Optional: Ear-Closing Pose

(1 minute or more)
My boat of life floats lightly
on tides of peace.

13. Fish Pose
(30 seconds)
My soul floats on waves
of cosmic light.

14. Supine Twist
(30–60 seconds to each side)
I open to the flow of
God's life within me.

15. Deep Relaxation in
the Corpse Pose
(5 minutes or more)
Bones, muscles, movement
I surrender now;
anxiety, elation and depression,
churning thoughts—
all these I give
into the hands of peace.

Medical Bibliography

Pruitt, A.A. (2000). Approach to the Patient with Headache. *Primary Care Medicine, Office Evaluation and Management of the Adult Patient, Fourth Edition.* Lippincott, Williams, and Wilkins.

Murphy, M, and Donovan, S. (1997). *The Physical and Psychological Effects of Meditation, Second Edition.* Institute of Noetic Sciences.

Robbins, L, and Lang, S. (2000). *Headache Help.* Houghton Mifflin Company.

Silberstein, S. et. al. (1998). *Headache in Clinical Practice.* Isis Medical Media.

Silberstein, S. et. al. (2000). Practice Parameter: Evidence-Based Guidelines for Migraine Headache (an Evidence-Based Review). *Neurology,* 55: 754–763.

Holroyd, K. et. al. (2001). Management of Chronic Tension-Type Headache with Tricyclic Antidepressant Medication, Stress Management Therapy, and Their Combination: A Randomized Controlled Trial. *JAMA,* 285: 2208–2215.

Goldberg, H. (1999). Feverfew for the Prevention of Migraine. *Alternative Medicine Alert,* 2: 41–43.

Kattapong, V. (2000). Biofeedback as a Treatment for Migraine. *Alternative Medicine Alert,* 3: 20–22.

Forker, A. (2001). Acupuncture for Migraine Headaches. *Alternative Medicine Alert,* 4: 31–34.

Ernst E. (1999). Homeopathic Prophylaxis of Headaches and Migraine? A Systematic Review. *Journal of Pain Symptom Management,* 18: 353–357.

Hoodin F., et al. (2000). Behavioral Self-Management in an Inpatient Headache Treatment Unit: Increasing Adherence and Relationship to Changes in Affective Distress. *Headache,* 40: 377–383.

De Leon, D. (1998). The Relaxation Response in the Treatment of Chronic Pain. *Alternative Medicine Alert,* 1: 13–16.

Whitlock, K. (2002). Drugs May Not Be Best Weapon against Teen Migraines, Study Finds. *Office of Research Communications, Ohio University.* News Release.

Richardson, K. (2002). Small Amounts of Deadly Toxin Proving Successful at Preventing Headaches. *Wake Forest University Baptist Medical Center.* News Release.

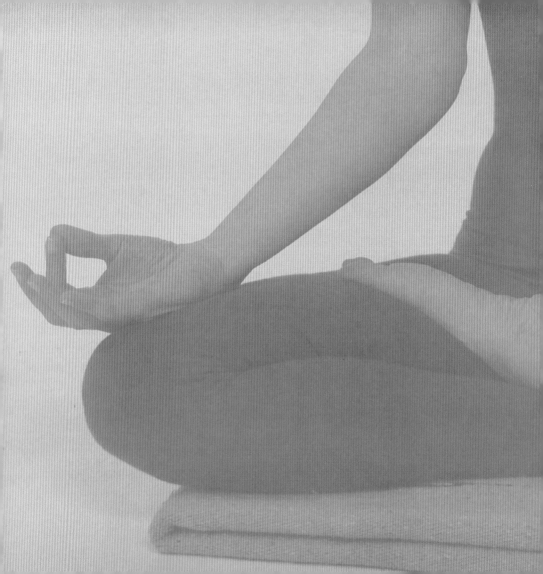

Additional Steps You Can Take with Ananda Yoga

At some point, you will be ready to begin practicing a more complete Ananda Yoga routine that will not only help prevent headaches and relieve stress, but bring your entire body and mind into greater harmony. You can increase the benefits of the postures even more by adding the practice of meditation, the central technique of all yoga.

To help you move in these directions, we recommend the resources below. The books and videos can be found at many bookstores or through:

Crystal Clarity Publishers

800-424-1055 or 530-478-7600

website: www.crystalclarity.com

Books

Ananda Yoga™ for Higher Awareness
Swami Kriyananda

This is the definitive book on Ananda Yoga™, by its founder. In addition to teaching a wide range of yoga postures, it offers breathing exercises and sample routines.

The Art and Science of Raja Yoga
Swami Kriyananda

This book/CD set includes everything in *Ananda Yoga for Higher Awareness*, plus many of the main aspects of the broader science of yoga, including philosophy, meditation, diet, and health.

How to Meditate
John Jyotish Novak

This book outlines the basics of meditation, including a classical yoga meditation technique.

Meditation for Starters,
Swami Kriyananda

This book/CD combination is an introduction to meditation; CD includes a guided meditation practice.

Videos

Yoga for Busy People
Gyandev McCord and Lisa Powers.

This video offers three 25-minute Ananda Yoga™ routines, one each for developing vitality, calmness, and harmonizing the heart.

Yoga for Emotional Healing
Lisa Powers

This video describes the basics of the Ananda Yoga™ approach to working with emotions, then offers a 45-minute practice routine.

Yoga to Awaken the Chakras
Gyandev McCord

This video describes the workings of the chakras (subtle energy centers within you), and how to use Ananda Yoga™ to work with the chakras to raise your consciousness.

Meditation Therapy for Stress & Change
Jyotish Novak

How to use meditation practices for dealing with the inevitable stresses and changes that life brings.

Meditation Therapy for Health and Healing
Jyotish Novak

How to use meditation practices for maintaining and restoring health, vitality, and harmony on all levels.

Music

Surrender: Mystical Music for Yoga
Derek Bell & Agni

More than just beautiful background music, the instrumental selections on *Surrender* are chosen and arranged to mirror the normal progression of yoga routines. Release tension, enter states of deep relaxation, and heighten your awareness. Can also be used to accompany healing work or meditation.

I, Omar

Donald Walters

Inspired by the ancient mystical poem The Rubaiyat of Omar Khayyam, this beautiful melody is taken up in turn by English horn, oboe, flute, harp, guitar, cello, violin, and strings. A favorite for yoga teachers and students alike.

Music to Awaken Superconsciousness

Donald Walters

Beautiful instrumental music designed to help the listener more easily access higher states of awareness, unlock intuitive guidance, and feel deep, lasting inner peace. Keyboards, harp, cello, violin, tamboura, and other instruments combine to create an utterly enchanting listening experience that will leave you feeling relaxed, uplifted, and inspired.

Relax: Meditations for Flute & Cello

Sharon Brooks & David Eby

This recording takes you on a journey deep within, helping you to experience a dynamic sense of peace and calmness. Relax is specifically designed to slow respiration and heart rate, bringing listeners to their calm center. The recording features fifteen melodies on flute and cello, accompanied by harp, guitar, keyboard, and strings.

Personal Training

The Expanding Light retreat is the primary teaching center for Ananda Yoga™ and Ananda Sangha, the spiritual work of which Ananda Yoga™ is a part. Located in the beautiful Sierra Nevada foothills of Northern California, the retreat is open year-round and offers programs in Ananda Yoga™, meditation, meditation therapy, health and healing, therapeutic yoga, yoga and meditation teacher training, silent retreats, self discovery, and much more.

For a free brochure,

call: 800-346-5350/530-478-7518

email: info@expandinglight.org

or visit: www.expandinglight.org

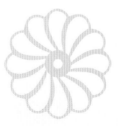